American Medical Association
Physicians dedicated to the health of America

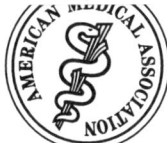

PRACTICE SUCCESS! SERIES

Managing Managed Care in the Medical Practice

The Physician's Handbook for Success and Survival

Project Manager/Editor: .... Kay Stanley
Project Assistant: .... Joyce Julian
Project Contributor:
Lauretta Mink, CMA, CMM
Art Director: .... Jeff Weir

Published by:

Coker Publishing, LLC —
in affiliation with The Coker Group
3150 Holcomb Bridge Road, Suite 200
Norcross, Georgia 30071
(770) 242-0118

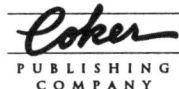

ISBN 0-89970-757-2

©1996 Coker Publishing, LLC

All contents of this book were compiled and written by The Coker Group and published by Coker Publishing, LLC, Norcross, Georgia. This book is under copyright. The materials herein may be reproduced for use by the purchaser; they may not be duplicated or distributed for commercial use without written permission from the publisher.

American Medical Association Preface

This book and the others contained in the *PRACTICE SUCCESS!*© Series are designed to offer you concrete, practical information on topics that you may sometimes consider the least important aspect of the profession of medicine: the business of running a medical practice. And in some ways that's how it should be. The long, hard years you dedicated to medical school and residency training were meant to make you an excellent physician, not an excellent businessperson. Caring for patients is and always will be your first priority. But you cannot successfully run a medical practice without planning and without consideration of important business issues. While it takes a minimum of ten years for a person to become a physician, the day a practice opens is the day a physician becomes a small businessperson.

Your many years of superb education probably did not include much information on medical office operations, personnel management, accounting or business law. Yet these business issues are more important than ever before, because the practice of medicine in today's rapidly changing environment is far more complex than ever before. Good business management today is essential to good medical practice. The physician who ignores basic business principles in operating his or her practice may soon find that they face difficulties with suppliers, employees, the government or even their patients.

Other pressures today force physicians to search for more efficient ways of running their practices. Most physicians find demands on their time increasing tremendously. There is a daily struggle to build a practice that will earn a steady income, to schedule regular working hours, to deliver quality care to patients and to still have time for relaxation and family.

Developing an efficient practice that runs smoothly makes all of these goals attainable. The application of good business planning will enable you to spend more time on those things that are most important to you.

This book and the others in the *PRACTICE SUCCESS!*© Series are guides to medical practice management for the new physician and the established physician who wants to survey his or her practice with an eye toward improvement. These books will not provide you with solutions to every challenge that may arise in day-to-day practice. Our goal is to acquaint you with essential business principles and tools, as well as with some new approaches to managing your practice. The knowledge you acquire from this series can be supplemented by information you gather from talking with your colleagues and advisors. You will then be in a position to explore those ideas that promise to achieve the best results for your particular practice situation.

By providing the information in this book and others, the **American Medical Association (AMA)** is not endorsing any one management philosophy or method of delivering health care services. No one approach will meet the objectives of all physicians. Physicians and their staffs will have to decide for themselves what is the best way to manage their individual practices. This guide is published by the American Medical Association for educational purposes only. It is intended solely to provide general information on managed care to assist physicians in making decisions. It is not intended to constitute legal advice and should not be relied on as a source of legal advice. If legal advice is desired or needed, a licensed attorney should be consulted. Finally, this book does not enunciate **AMA** policy. The annual *Policy Compendium* of the **AMA** sets forth our positions on such issues as contracting, policy, medical ethics, managed care and practice management.

We hope that this publication will be useful to you.

The American Medical Association

About The Coker Group

The Coker Group is a national provider of health care consultative and management services assisting physicians, hospitals, and health care systems to better position themselves to be successful in a reformed health care environment. The Coker Group offers the following services for its clients:

Programs and Services:

- Primary Care Physician Network Development
- Practice Valuations and Acquisition Negotiations
- Physician Employment and Compensation Contract Design
- The Facilitation of Group Practice Development
- Physician Practice Management Services
- Management Services Organization (MSO) Development
- Market Share Management Program
- Newly Recruited Physician Services
- Educational Programs
- Evaluation and Consultant Services
- Personnel Productivity Programs
- *PRACTICE SUCCESS!*© and *PRACTICE SUCCESS!*© Series

For more information, contact:

THE Coker GROUP
National Consultants to Healthcare Providers

The Coker Group / 3150 Holcomb Bridge Road / Suite 200
Norcross, Georgia 30071 / (770) 242-0118

About The Book

Managing Managed Care in the Medical Practice addresses one of the most challenging issues encountered in medical practice management in this decade: how to understand, assess, and evaluate managed care arrangements offered in the marketplace. Virtually every medical practice in the United States today is faced with daily decisions about managed care.

Health care reform has pressured physicians to make decisions to participate, or not to participate, in complex plans offered by insurers. Plans range from government programs such as Medicare and Medicaid to those offered by traditional indemnity companies. On the scene, also, are programs offered by hospitals and physician alliances. The survival of the medical practice may depend on the decisions made regarding plan participation. This book attempts to lay a foundation for making sound decisions about managed care contracts.

The information contained in *Managing Managed Care in the Medical Practice* is meant to provide physicians and others with the basic tools necessary to survive and thrive in managed care markets. It combines information from a variety of sources and regions of the country. This information should serve as a supplemental guideline only and is not meant to substitute for the advise of an attorney, business or financial planner.

Who should read this book?

This book is a direct, single-topic guide to understanding managed care for those involved in the "business side of medicine," including:

- practicing physicians
- owners of medical practices and clinics
- practice administrators and managers
- business managers of any medical business
- business administrators in health care facilities, nursing homes, or health agencies

Anyone interested in the "how to" aspects of evaluating managed care agreements would benefit from this information.

What information can the reader find?

The reader will find practical and specific information and formulas for use in the day-to-day operation of the medical practice, including:

- What do these managed care terms mean?
- What are the advantages and disadvantages of participation?
- How do I develop a managed care strategy that fits my organization?
- What do I need to know about reimbursement under capitation?
- How do I analyze a managed care contract?

- How do I determine and redetermine the plan's effectiveness?
- How does this impact my practice or organization?
- How does managed care affect ethical concerns?
- How do I market in a managed care environment?

How technical is the writing?

Managing Managed Care in the Medical Practice is written in an informal, practical style. There are few terms in this handbook that are not found regularly in a newspaper, and there are no discussions that would appear out-of-place in a business memorandum. This publication is a nontechnical discussion about managing managed care as it relates to medical practice management.

About the Contributors

Special appreciation and acknowledgement is extended to the following project participants:

J. Harper Gaston, MD, President and Chief Executive Officer of Healthcare Partnership Consultants, Inc., Greenville, GA, he has had over thirty years of leadership experience with Kaiser Permanente and other health care organizations.

Dr. Gaston has developed, successfully negotiated and implemented an innovative approach to capitation and a detailed financial model for capitation contracts. Over the last eight years he has been a strong advocate of creating a physician group without walls concept. This strategy has been successfully implemented with hundreds of community-based physicians in four major cities in the Southeast.

Dr. Gaston receive his B.S. in Medicine from Emory University in 1952 and his M.D. in 1955. He is certified by the Board of Internal Medicine and was elected to AOA in 1983 by the Emory University School of Medicine. He served as Assistant Clinical Professor of Medicine at Stanford University from 1971 to 1977 and was on the Medical Advisory Committee of Chabot College from 1967 to 1977. He currently serves as a member of the Advisory Council for the Emory University School of Medicine.

Anne Renz, Vice President, Allina Health System, Minneapolis, MN, has been active in the health care field for over twenty years, beginning her career as a registered nurse. She has twice served as a hospital CEO for ten years of her career, actively guided a hospital merger and held a variety of administrative positions in predecessor organizations to the Allina Health System. Her current role involves providing administration for the Professional Services Group of Allina which provides the linkage between physicians and the System and houses the departments of Graduate Medical Education, Continuing Medical Education, Physician Recruitment, Medical Policy, Physician Support Services, Research, Tele-medicine and the Allina Medical Group. In addition, she serves as the senior human resources executive to all of Allina s fifty-plus clinics and its employed complement of over five hundred providers.

A national speaker and author of several articles, Ms. Renz also provides occasional consulting services in areas of physician recruitment, managed care issues and multiple administrative concerns.

Roland E. Deaton, Jr., MBA, is a member of the Health Care Services Group of G.R. Rush & Company, P.C., Chattanooga, TN. Mr. Deaton has fifteen years of health care management experience, having held various management positions in the health care industry. Deaton earned an MHA in Health and Hospital Administration and is a Certified Public Accountant.

Other contributors include Lauretta Mink, David Webb, CPA, and other members of The Coker Group staff.

Managing Managed Care in the Medical Practice is based on a section excerpt from a 500+ page medical practice management resource entitled *PRACTICE SUCCESS!*© Introduced in 1993, this textbook has ongoing updates and enhancements. As publishers, we are committed to providing the most current information concerning topics of interest for the "business side of medicine." For more information on this and other resources available, contact:

Coker Publishing, LLC
3150 Holcomb Bridge Road
Suite 200
Norcross, GA 30071
(770) 242-0118

Managing Editor
Kay B. Stanley

Overview

As health care reform advances, it is inevitable that every physician will be involved with some form of managed care. Generally, we think of managed care as any formal arrangement between physicians, hospitals, and a non-provider third party with fees and utilization standards to provide the highest quality care possible to patients, within agreed upon cost restraints.

Managed care plans continue to evolve, with features from one plan appearing in others and new features being developed. The topics in this book will enable you to function in a managed care environment by providing you the following information:

- Fundamentals and concepts, including terminology and definitions
- Clarification of various roles of physicians in managed care, their relationships and interactions
- Tools for assessing plans and reviewing contracts
- Methods for measuring payment effectiveness and impact on your practice
- Patterns for cost-effective health care management
- Explanations of capitation payment systems
- Strategies for capitation issues and approaches
- Tactics for positioning your practice in the managed care marketplace
- Current state of Medicare and Medicaid in managed care

Table of Contents

Chapter 1 — Managed Care Basics 1

Understanding the Concept 3
How Does it Work? 4
Advantages and Disadvantages of Participation 5
Terminology 7
Descriptions 7
Terms and Definitions 12

Chapter 2 — Physician Roles in Managed Care 25

The Role of the Primary Care Physician 25
    Qualities and Capabilities of a Personal Care Manager 27
    Management Tools 27
The Role of the Nonprimary Care Physician Specialist 28
Qualities and Capabilities of a Specialist 29
    Management Tools 29

Chapter 3 — Developing a Managed Care Strategy 31

Assessing Your Practice 31
Assessing Proposed Contracts 31
Assessing the Effectiveness of Existing Contracts 32
Assessing the Current Practice 32
Financial Information 32
Practice Geographic and Demographic Information 32
Practice Capacity and Capabilities 33
Assessing Proposed Contracts 33
    General Plan Information 33
    Financial Information 33
    Employer/Employee Information 33
    Obtain References from Current Participants 34
Managed Care Contract Review Steps 34

Chapter 4 — Assessing the Impact on Your Practice 41

Practice Capacity 41
Patient Source Analysis 42
Service Analysis 43
Cost Analysis 44

Chapter 5 — Payment Effectiveness of a Managed Care Contract 47

How Payment Effective is the Managed Care Plan 48
Re-evaluate the Managed Care Plan 51

Chapter 6 — Cost-Effective Health Care 53

Physician Education: The Key to Promoting Cost-Effective Care 53
Practice Guidelines 54
Information Sharing 54
Economic Analysis 55
Medical Resource Management 56
Outcomes Measurement 56

Chapter 7 — Capitation Payment Systems 57

Basic Capitation 59
Risk Pools 61
Withholds and Bonus Payments 63
Accounting for Expenses Incurred but Not Reported 63
Carve-outs 63
Capitation for Subspecialists 64
Percentage of Premium Reimbursement 64
Copayments and Deductibles 64

Chapter 8 — Capitation Strategies 65

Capitation Strategies — Multiple Issues, Multiple Approaches 65
Capitation Strategies — Another View 67

Chapter 9 — Determining Reimbursement 71

Here's What You Need to Compare 71
Determine the Weighted Average of the Plan 72

Chapter 10 — Marketing to the Managed Care Marketplace 75

Positioning in the Marketplace 75
    Practice Evaluation and Assessment 76
    Marketing to Payers and Employers 76
    Marketing in Managed Care 77
    Concentrate on Patient Satisfaction 77
Know Your Contract — Down to the Last Clause 78
Adjust Your Appointment Schedule to Protect the Practice 78
Reach Out with Mid-Level Providers 78
Use the Telephone — Effectively 79
Take "No" for an Answer 80
Document and Demonstrate Patient Satisfaction 81
Who is Marketing What to Whom? 81
Tips to Market Your Practice and Increase Patient Satisfaction 82
How to Use a Patient Satisfaction Survey 84
How to Handle an Audit by a Managed Care Organization 84

Chapter 11 — A Word about Medicare and Medicaid 87

Medicare Contracts 87
In Capitation, Prevention Pays 88
Case Management Helps Minimize the Risk 88

Chapter 12 — Ethical Considerations in Managed Care 91

The Physician-Patient Relationship 91
    Conflicts Between Physician and Patient 92
    Patient Autonomy Responsibility 92
Guidelines 93

AMA Principles of Managed Care 97

Exhibits 103

Determine the Weighted Average of the Plan (Schedule A) 105
Determine the Weighted Average of the Plan (Schedule B) 107
Patient Satisfaction Survey 109

Bibliography 111

Index 113

Managed Care Basics

Managed care is difficult to define due to its evolving nature, but in general terms it is "the process of managing costs" through the efficiency and effectiveness of delivering care. It does not translate to poor care when done well, but equates to streamlining the system so that patients receive appropriate care in the appropriate setting at the least cost possible.

The National Association of Children's Hospitals has defined managed care as:

> *An attempt to contain health care costs by controlling how and where patients obtain health care services. Any health insurance or health financing control mechanism or financial inducement intended to direct or restrict the patient's choice of provider or the patient/physician's choice of treatment modality.*

Physicians who work in managed care may argue that truly effective managed care focuses on managing care rather than managing cost. In the book *The Physician and Managed Care*, written by David E. Vogel, published by the American Medical Association, managed care is defined as follows:

> *A means of providing health care services within a defined network of health care providers who are given the responsibility to manage and provide high quality, cost-effective health care to a defined population.*

Edward F.X. Hughes, M.D., MPH, J.L. Kellogg Graduate School of Management and The Center for Health Services and Policy Research, Northwestern University, Evanston, Illinois in the book *The Physician's Guide to Managed Care*, edited by David B. Nash and published by Aspen Publishers offers this definition:

> *Managed care is the process of the application of standard business practices to the delivery of health care in the traditions of the American free enterprise system.*

Lastly, the American Society of Internal Medicine (ASIM) defines managed care as:

> *A system of health care delivery through contracted providers in which the entities responsible for financing the cost of health care exert influence on the clinical decision-making of those who provide health care in an attempt to provide health care which is cost-effective, accessible, and of acceptable quality.*

Distinguishing features of managed care include: (i) a network of contracted providers; (ii) the channeling of patients to contracted providers through limitations on benefits to those insureds who use non-contracting providers; (iii) some type of utilization management and quality assurance systems; and (iv) a shifting of the financial risk to the providers of health care.

The debate over definition will continue. The importance of looking at the system in place or as proposed for the patients you serve will be the most important place to focus your energy. There will, in all likelihood, never be "one" managed care definition, but rather multiple variations on the theme.

Statistically speaking:

- 20 percent of the U.S. population is covered by a Health Maintenance Organization (HMO) plan;

- 63 percent of employees covered by a health plan are enrolled in an HMO or other form of managed care;

- Of the 33,634,000 people enrolled in Medicaid in 1994, 23.2 percent (7,794,250) were in an HMO or other form of managed care, up from 9.5 percent (2,696,397 out of 28,280,000) in 1991;

- Average cost per worker covered is $3,485 for HMOs versus $3,850 for traditional indemnity coverage;

- Patient satisfaction ranges from more than 75 percent in the top-rated plans to less than 35 percent in the lowest rated HMO.

Sources: *U.S. Dept. of Health and Human Services; Group Health Association of America; CareData Reports, Inc.; Foster Higgins.*

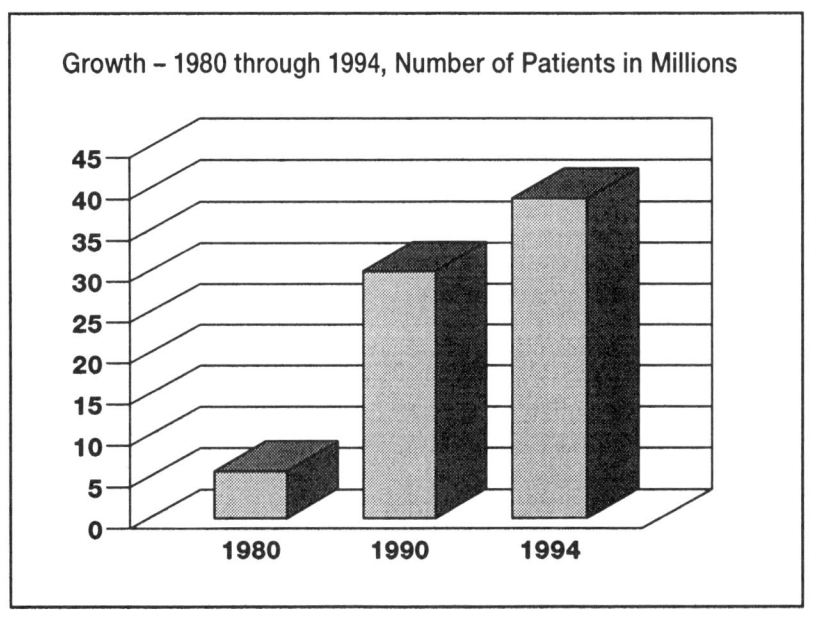

HMO Enrollment

Growth – 1980 through 1994, Number of Patients in Millions

> *"It must be remembered
> that there is nothing more difficult to plan,
> more doubtful of success,
> nor more dangerous to manage,
> than the creation of a new system.
> For the initiator has the enmity
> of all who would profit
> by the preservation of the old institutions
> and meekly lukewarm defenders
> in those who would gain by the new ones."*
>
> — Niccoló Machiavelli

Managed care—the term is not new. Physicians have been managing care and expectations of patients and family members for centuries. Since time began, they have been managing illness. They have sought ways to build and change the systems to better treat disease, and the social and economic ravages it places on the lives of their patients and society. So why, in the 1990's does the term "managed care" become so concerning, so controversial and so debatable?

The managed care systems we have begun to build in the past fifteen years have not concentrated primarily on disease and prevention, but on ways to organize the system, to create or restrict access and to finance the care of millions. It has been spreading fast—leaving a trail of successes and failures in its wake. We are in the midst of building something new—of integrating the care management with the financial management and attempting to strike a balance where neither suffers and the doctor-patient relationship prevails. This is an onerous task that calls upon physicians to demonstrate outstanding business and care management skills. It is also one that calls upon administrators to seek to collaborate and not to control. And it is one that, in general, calls for an integration of talents to a degree that the health care industry has not seen in its rich history.

The journey has begun. Those who are in health care—either as provider, payer or consumer, will be part of designing the trip and determining the destination, regardless of an active or passive role. You are involved. You will contribute and this contribution should not be underestimated. Your task is to decide how and what difference you will make.

Understanding the Concept

From a physician's perspective, managed care is:

> *A process that involves managing patients, referrals, admissions, discharges, ancillary service, resources, and outcomes. The primary responsibility for clinical decision-making remains with the physician.*

To be successful, managed care organizations must focus on supporting the physician clinical decision-making process. Similarly, the primary focus of physicians in successful managed care organizations (MCOs) must be on the doctor-patient interface and the clinical processes that occur there.

Physicians must be proactive in health-care reform by managing patients, resources, and outcomes. Otherwise, MCOs, insurance companies, and government will artificially control cost and utilization by controlling access, discounting fees, and implementing price controls. These are clearly undesirable options, primarily because they impose administrative interventions upon the doctor-patient relationship.

The objectives of managed care are: (1) to maximize quality; (2) to maximize patient service; and (3) to minimize total costs per person per year. By accomplishing these objectives, physicians and MCOs increase the value of the health care service they are providing to their patients and members. By increasing value, providers and MCOs meet patient and payer (market) demands. It only stands to reason that market-driven and value-based providers and MCOs have the greatest likelihood of being rewarded with a steady flow of patients.

How Does it Work?

In its most basic sense, managed care works by reducing overutilization. As an example, MCOs have focused on reducing the number of hospital days utilized. This is accomplished by conducting preadmission testing, concurrent utilization review, second surgical opinion, same day surgery, home care, and case management. These techniques have contributed to a continued steady decline in hospital days utilized — a trend expected to continue throughout the 1990's, and beyond.

Physician office services and hospital outpatient services are the current utilization targets for many MCOs. Techniques to control this utilization typically include case management requirements, drug formularies, practice management support systems/guidelines and referral authorizations for subspecialty, ancillary, and other nonprimary care services.

Objectives also may be achieved through defined provider networks; benefits design, such as coverage limitations and expansions; cost sharing through copayments, coinsurance, and deductibles; provider incentive/risk-sharing systems; quality management systems; and management information systems.

Definitions of managed care are reliant on the "philosophy" of the MCO, its providers, and the major purchasers (employers, federal and state government). These "perspectives" serve as driving forces in the process. The first force drives from those who see this process as an opportunity "to do it better." This is the professional force. The second force is comprised of those who see this process as an opportunity to make money. This is the economic force. The two are linked and yet often at odds with each other in MCOs. These forces are translated into MCO organizational structure, quality and utilization systems design and operation, provider incentive system design, and other "infrastructure" factors. Therefore, it is important for the physician comparing or evaluating an MCO to objectively determine which perspective (or driving force) prevails.

It is important to clarify who is "managing" the care: the MCO or the primary care physicians and the subspecialists to whom they refer? A primary function of the well-run MCO is to provide support and an infrastructure that furnishes physicians the tools that enable them to better manage care. An examination of the MCO and discussions regarding actual case management will provide insight into how well this is being managed.

Successful managed care requires interdependence between the MCO and its physicians. To achieve quality and cost objectives, MCOs are dependent on the quality of physicians they recruit. Similarly, no physician can manage care effectively without substantial support from the MCO. The relationship must facilitate an equally beneficial partnership.

Advantages and Disadvantages of Participation

As with any business opportunity, there are both the "pros" and "cons" in participating in managed care plans. The advantages often seem readily apparent while the disadvantages are often more obscure. With the multitude of managed care organizations in the United States, the physician may be confused as he or she discovers the wide variations that exist among them. A physician's decision to participate, or with which organizations to contract, is not an easy one. Below, we offer an outline of considerations that may be useful in the sorting process.

In considering *advantages*:

- **Increase in patient base**
    - What will be the potential increase in the size of the patient base?
    - What is the mix? (Age, gender, risk status, etc.)
    - What is the length of the contract?
    - Can I accommodate this increase without adding additional staff? If I add staff, what will happen when this contract expires?

- **Guaranteed capitated income based on number of covered lives regardless of the number of visits**
    - Can/will I (or my group) be able to control utilization?
    - Does the plan provide any assistance in wellness programs or will I need to offer that to decrease the visits to my practice?
    - What are the health risks associated with this patient population?
    - How have other physicians in this plan generally fared under this capitated level?
    - What are the enrollees being told about access to care? Are they being encouraged to visit often for prevention? Are there copays for this plan and are they at a level that encourages preventive care instead of encouraging patients to delay care?
    - Will we need to expand clinic hours to meet patient demand?

- **Prevention of patient migration to other physicians who participate in this plan**
    - How often can patients change primary care providers?
    - What other physicians are in this plan?
    - How competitive is my practice in attracting patients (e.g., is it conveniently located, are the hours of operation conducive to this patient population, is it attractive, are the patient satisfaction surveys to date complimentary, is the staff cordial, etc.)?

In considering *disadvantages*:

- **Increase in practice expense**
    - What will the increased practice expense be to accommodate this patient base?
    - Will I need to add more support staff to handle precertification, case management and the data demands of the plan?
    - Is my staff able to help with patient management difficulties? What education might they require?

- **Decreased revenue per potential patient**
  - What payment method is the MCO using?
  - How much Medicare and Medicaid business will come to my practice and at what rate of payment?
  - Is the volume going to accommodate for the downward pressure on the use of ancillary services?

- **Accounts receivable days**
  - Will I have to wait longer for reimbursement due to increased administrative effort in my office?
  - Will utilization restrictions and the accompanying review time delay my payments?
  - What is the average time from claim submission to payment?
  - What is the experience of some of my colleagues under this plan?

- **Liability and malpractice exposure**
  - Will I see an increase in exposure? What experiences have my colleagues had?
  - What is the general experience of the plan in this area?
  - What happens when I have a clinical decision conflict with the MCO? Who do I talk to and what are the appeal options?
  - Who else is in the plan? To whom do I have to make referrals and how well do I know them?
  - How and how often does the plan update me on changes in participating physicians?
  - What about patients in the plan who are currently under the care of a specialist who is not in the plan? Is there any "Grandfathering?" If so, who bears the financial risk?

- **Potential loss of a large group of patients with plan changes**
  - On what grounds can the plan exclude me after I have signed a contract?
  - If one physician from our group is excluded, what happens to the rest of us regarding call, cross coverage, general plan participation, etc.?
  - What is the length of the enrollee contract?
  - What is the plan's experience in retaining contracts year to year?
  - How will my group be marketed in this plan?
  - What is the length of the termination notice?

- **Data requirements**
  - What data will I need to submit initially and continuously to participate?
  - Will this add to my administrative overhead?
  - What happens to this data? Who has access to it and will I be notified?
  - Is data collected to be used in an educational or punitive manner?

Answers to all these questions (and more depending upon the initial findings) will be essential in determining the "fit" between your practice and the MCO. Do not short cut the due diligence process in making your decisions. Be sure to speak with colleagues who are in the plan or who have opted to not join. Seek their perspectives in this decision.

Terminology

To understand the basics of managed care, one must become familiar with acronyms, organization descriptions, and plan terminology commonly encountered. "Provider" refers generically to individuals and organizations involved in providing care to patients. "Members" or "covered lives" refers to individuals or patients who receive, or are eligible to receive care.

EPO	Exclusive Provider Organization
GPWW	Group Practice Without Walls
HMO	Health Maintenance Organization
IDS	Integrated Delivery System
IPA	Independent Physicians Association
MCO	Managed Care Organization
MSO	Management Service Organization
PHO	Physician-Hospital Organization
POS	Point of Service Plan
PPO	Preferred Provider Organization
TOP	Triple Option Plan

Descriptions

Differences in managed care organizations are becoming blurred as new systems take pieces of current systems and blend them. The brief descriptions below begin to describe the systems of today. Change will be constant. One must be judicious in examining each plan for its terms and not relying on a "label" to provide a full, clear description.

Exclusive Provider Organization (EPO). A variation of the Preferred Provider Organization (PPO), EPOs provide one level of benefits. While the patient is still able to select a physician/hospital from the panel of network providers, there is no coverage for going out of network. (Note: Most plans have a provision for emergency care when one is traveling out of the area.) Due to the restriction to these exclusive providers, EPO premiums can be priced to compete more closely with HMOs, yet maintain some of the freedom of choice of the PPO. EPOs are often the result of employers working with savvy health care purchasers and selecting their own network of hospitals and providers. The plan functions on limiting administrative costs. Premiums can also be set on the experience of the employee group and not on a community rating, thus "tailoring" the plan to the company's employee base needs. Another term for this arrangement is EPA— Exclusive Provider Arrangements.

Group Practice Without Walls (GPWW). In a Group Practice Without Walls, physicians align to contract with managed care companies as a group. The key to the success of this plan is strong alignment and centralizing administrative functions while maintaining independent office locations. Legal and financial requirements for forming a GPWW vary by region. They should be thoroughly investigated before deciding to form this type of entity. Additionally, reduction of administrative costs and centralization of administrative functions often means staff in individual offices must be relocated or not retained. The political and financial consequences of these decisions should be thoroughly examined. If the groups are unwilling to reduce their administrative overhead, they will not maximize the benefit of this arrangement.

Health Maintenance Organizations (HMOs). HMOs function in a variety of ways, but all function in a federally regulated environment. The variances lie in the methods of delivering care, but many characteristics are common. They contract with a network of providers (physicians, hospitals and others) to deliver care to a defined population of enrollees. HMOs provide individual participants with "packaged" health care services in exchange for a fixed monthly premium —"prepaid" health care. Like insurance companies, HMOs accept premiums in exchange for financing the cost of covered medical care. Like a health care delivery system, they arrange to provide care either directly or by contract. Contracts are set with a restricted set of providers and hospitals for a prearranged period. They hold down health care costs by transferring significant portions of the economic risk to providers and limiting the number of approved services. Care to the enrollee is monitored by the HMO through the following process:

- precertifying elective procedures and certain tests
- formally reviewing ongoing hospitalizations (concurrent review)
- planning for the discharge of the patient at the onset of hospitalization, and
- determining what services would enable the patient to leave the acute care hospital earlier to be cared for in a more appropriate setting (e.g., at home with home care services, nursing home for rehabilitation, etc.) and systematically managing each case.

HMOs have medical directors and a team of professionals to provide these services. There is also an appeals plan if the physician and/or patient does not feel the care or decisions are appropriate.

Though the models are continually changing, there are six that commonly are recognized as of this writing. In contracting with HMOs, physicians should weigh these points (advantages and disadvantages) and what effect they will have on the practice. There are three viewpoints to consider: the physician's, the HMO's and the patient's. It is unlikely that advantages and disadvantages will be equal to each of the three players in every scenario.

- **Staff Model.** Physicians are salaried employees, although there may be outside contracts for some medical specialty or medical consultant services.

  Advantages:
  - HMO has a high degree of control over physicians that increases control over utilization;
  - Patients may experience convenience in that facilities generally are located in one place.

  Disadvantages:
  - HMO experiences significant costs in developing the infrastructure and the need to pay salaries to staff physicians regardless of patient volumes;
  - Patients have a limited choice of physicians and, if they are not proximate to the care delivery site, may not find the facility location convenient.

- **Group Practice Model.** This model revolves around a multispecialty group of independent physicians providing services to contracted members. These physicians may also be permitted to see members of other HMOs or non-HMO patients. This model is used in states that prohibit the employment of physicians by non-physicians (the Corporate Practice of Medicine).

Advantages:

- Fees can be generated by seeing non-HMO patients to offset salary and administrative expenses;
- Patients can experience "one-stop shopping" and a strongly coordinated system of care.

Disadvantages:

- Depending upon the size of the enrollee base, the HMO may comprise only a small portion of the practice and may not have as much "clout" with the physician group;
- Patients' choice in provider selection is limited.

- **Network Model.** The HMO contracts with several physicians or physician groups to provide services, securing a network to meet the demographic and geographic needs of the enrollee base. This network includes selected hospital and outpatient service sites.

Advantages:

- HMO can include broader participation among physicians in the community;
- Patients have a wide choice of physicians and facility locations.

Disadvantages:

- Larger physician base limits the volume and thus the amount of influence the HMO can exert over any one physician or physician group;
- The HMO must screen and credential many providers, often limiting the statistical analysis that can be applied to physicians who are seeing minimum number of patients for the plan;
- When the plan has a large physician base, the referral sources are varied and there is often a problem with providing care continuity from one specialist to another.

- **Independent Practice Association (IPA)-Type Model.** This model utilizes (generally) multiple corporations formed by physicians who are each maintaining their practices. They participate in an Independent Practice Association in order to secure managed care business and provide a vehicle for accepting financial risk for members through capitation or discounted fees. This model provides good positioning for physicians to assume the responsibility for providing care to members in exchange for a fixed amount per member each month. The risks are spread throughout the IPA. It also offers a variety of physician compensation mechanisms. Generally, specialists are on a discounted fee-for-service basis and primary care physicians are on an individual capitated basis.

Advantages:

- Capital requirements for the HMO are low because the associations and administrative systems are already in place.
- Physicians are in an organized entity to deal with the HMO which translates into stronger financial and policy setting power;
- Physicians retain outside practices and have separate sources of income including participation in multiple other managed care plans;
- The autonomous physician organization can often have greater influence over clinical decision making when they are separate from the HMO and have a base of business that is not dependent upon only one managed care plan.
- Patients have a broad choice of participating physicians who are practicing in private offices.

Disadvantages:

- Depending upon the volume of patients and the length of the contract, a substantial portion of the practice's business can change with any given plan year change;
- Participation in multiple managed care plans places administrative burdens on the practice to submit data specific to each plan.

- **Direct Contract Model.** In this model, the HMO contracts directly with a panel of physicians, relying heavily on primary care physicians. These physicians act as care managers (or gatekeepers) for delivery of direct services and assumption of responsibility for making referrals to specialists. Each physician on the panel bargains independently with the HMO as an individual or through his or her small group practice.

  Advantages:
  - Physicians maintain maximum autonomy;
  - The network is easily configured to meet the geographic needs of the enrollees.

  Disadvantages:
  - Model does not furnish an organized negotiating vehicle for participating physicians;
  - Utilization management is more difficult because physicians participate on an individual or small group basis.

- **Specialty HMO Models.** In these models, the HMO is contracting in one area of medical specialty, such as orthopedics or obstetrics to provide prepaid coverage to its members. These models are often set on a discounted fee-for-service basis.

Integrated Delivery Systems (IDS). An IDS is a seamless consolidation of providers (hospitals, physicians, etc.) that focuses on the coordination, delivery, and management of care to a defined population.

- Among the variations noted in the evolving marketplace:
  - *Community Integrated Delivery System (CIDS)*
  - *Provider Integrated Delivery System (PIDS)*

Independent Practice Association (IPA). An IPA is a corporation formed by physicians who maintain their independent practices but participate in the IPA to secure managed care business. IPAs accept financial risk for their members through capitation or discounted fees. The *group* is spread out geographically and is less formal than a group or staff model HMO. The only association between IPA providers is an individual contract between the physicians and the insurance company.

IPAs were originally formed to allow independent, community-based physicians a vehicle to compete with Staff and Group model HMOs. IPAs typically have a core of primary care physicians responsible for acting as *gatekeepers* (providing basic primary care and) by managing all medical services and authorizing all referrals to specialists. Experts disagree about the long-term success of an IPA to compete effectively against Staff and Group model providers due to the inherent efficiencies in these other models.

In today's marketplace, the distinction between IPAs and PPOs is blurred. PPOs are becoming more integrated by providing at least some administrative services. Independent IPAs, not associated with any specific HMO, but formed and controlled as a contracting vehicle by and for physicians, are becoming common.

Management Service Organization (MSO). An organization established to relieve the physicians of the administrative duties of running a practice while allowing them to retain ownership of their patient charts and records. The organization is set up either by physicians, a hospital, or an independent party and furnishes them to a professional corporation of physicians for a monthly service fee.

There can be an exclusive contract with one professional corporation or a contract with more than one professional corporation. The physicians in the professional corporation can be independent contractors, employees or partners in the corporation. The patient charts typically are retained by the physicians unless they are employees of the corporation.

Most MSOs of not-for-profit hospitals are for-profit subsidiaries. It is hard to qualify an MSO as not-for-profit. Two examples of MSOs are Alta Bates MSO in Berkeley, California, and Mullikan Medical Group in Orange County, California.

Physician-Hospital Organization (PHO). An organization structured traditionally with 50 percent control and ownership by physicians and 50 percent control and ownership by the hospital. PHOs are established to secure joint contracts with third party payers.

The term PHO is also generically used to represent many different types of physician and hospital relationships and integration models. PHOs are often seen as transitional models in that they can be the first organizing step for a medical staff or group of independent physicians. Traditionally, they have had difficulty moving to a model where a single signature can commit the entire group.

Point of Service Plan (POS). (Open HMO or Swing Plan) Point of Service Plans are based upon an HMO format. They demand the selection of a primary care physician, but allow for opting out of the network (called self-referring) at a substantially reduced benefit.

POS premiums generally are priced to be competitive with an HMO. They have the associated utilization management mechanisms, but also provide out-of-network flexibility, although generally at a significant financial expense to the physician member.

Preferred Provider Organization (PPO). PPOs are networks comprised of a panel of independent physicians that health insurance companies and health benefit plans contract with for health care services at a discounted fee.

This form of insurance typically contains two levels of benefits. The patient can choose his or her provider at the time services are needed/provided. The first level—provided within the PPO network of providers—provides the highest coverage, typically 90 to 100 percent of covered services. The second level—for services provided outside of the PPO network—still provides benefits, but typically at a minimum of 20 percent lower than the In-Network benefit. Sometimes these are called Double Option plans.

This difference provides a financial incentive to the patient to utilize preferred providers, thus enabling the insurance company to demonstrate channeled (or directed) business to a provider in exchange for a discount. This channeling effect, in addition to utilization review, limited drug formulary, preadmission authorization and other mechanisms, also contributes to managed care discounts.

Triple Option Plans (TOP). These types of insurance plans typically contain three levels of benefits, each with various levels of flexibility to the insured. As the level of flexibility increases, so does the amount the insured must pay out-of-pocket. These types of programs are also called step-down benefit plans.

An example is an HMO allowing the insured to self-select a PPO-type plan or an indemnity plan at increased amounts of out-of-pocket expense to the insured. In doing so, the insured has greater flexibility in the ability to choose a physician or a hospital and often will be less disrupted if an employer changes plans on an annual basis.

Terms and Definitions

The language of managed care is evolving. The next pages provide you with some useful terms and definitions that will be important to your understanding of the remainder of this text. Many terms are basic and will be familiar to you. Others are just emerging and are often more prevalent in one part of the country than another. Write down terms being used in your area for future reference and to help other colleagues as they enter the managed care arena in years to come.

Access
Potential and actual entry of a population into the health care delivery system. Elements of access include availability, affordability and approachability.

Accountable Health Plans (AHPs)
As proposed in the Clinton plan, AHPs are state-certified health plans and provider networks that include hospitals, primary care physicians, specialty care physicians, and other providers and sites that can offer a full range of preventive and treatment services. Accountability to the public and the populations served would have high priority. Many people use terms such as *Coordinated Care Network(s) (CCN), Integrated Health System (IHS), and Integrated Service Networks (ISNs) as substitutes for AHP.*

Accredited Capitated Provider (ACP)
A health care providing entity that (1) receives capitated payments from a community network under a contract to provide health services to the network's enrollees. A health care providing entity is capitated when its compensation arrangement with a network involves the provider's acceptance of material financial risk for the delivery of a predetermined set of services for a specified period; (2) is licensed to provide and provides the contracted services, either directly, or through an affiliate; (3) agrees to serve as an ACP of a community network to reduce the network's net worth and deposit requirements; (4) is approved by the commissioner of health; and (5) agrees to provide services without compensation to enrollees for an insolvent community network for up to 120 days after the network has been declared insolvent. A term first introduced in 1993 and further defined in Minnesota's 1994 health reform legislation. This term is also used in other parts of the country on a selective basis.

Actuarial Analysis
The application of probability and statistical methods to calculate risk of occurrence of events such as illness, hospitalization, disability or death. Health insurance companies use actuarial tools to project probable health service utilization and costs likely to be incurred for the lives they cover. These procedures use many differentiating factors (e.g., sex, age, employment status, location, family status, proximity to providers, etc.) which may be used to set premium rates for health insurance. The premium rates are intended to cover the claims expense and provide a profit margin.

Administrative Services Only (ASO)
An arrangement between a third-party insurance company and a self-funded plan sponsored by an employer where the third-party company performs administrative services only and does not assume any risks. The employer is at risk for the cost of health care services provided. Services may include claims processing, actuarial analysis, utilization review, data reporting, and stop-loss coverage.

All Payer System
A pricing system in which all providers and payers are forced to participate. Under an all payer system it is possible for a number of payers to exist, thereby maintaining a sense of *pluralism*. However, all payers pay the same for the same service, regardless of volume or other considerations.

Alternative Delivery Systems
Health care delivery modes that provide an alternative to traditional *fee-for-service* by integrating financing issues with patient care services. Anything done outside the inpatient setting or the physician's office based on a payment structure other than fee-for-service medicine used to be considered "alternative". However, today's rapidly changing health care environment with the growth of *IPAs, HMOs, PPOs* and other *managed care* entities, has made the "alternative" more like the norm. The shape of health care reform also indicates this trend will continue throughout the decade.

Alternative Primary Care Practitioner
These nonphysician care givers, such as nurse practitioners, midwives, physician assistants and extenders, provide *primary medical care* services at locations varying from rural health clinics to physician offices. The range of primary care services they can deliver is defined by state law as is the level of physician supervision they require. The current shortage of primary care physicians and the increased emphasis on primary care delivery demands that new ways and means of care provision be examined.

Ambulatory Care
Health care services provided to patients who are not inpatients of hospitals or other residential facilities (e.g., residential treatment centers, nursing homes). May include care provided to hospital outpatients.

Antitrust Laws
A group of statutes that outline fair trade practices in a competitive marketplace. The chief enforcer of these laws is the Federal Trade Commission (FTC). The FTC is a five-person administrative agency that conducts investigations, announces rules and regulations and enforces statutory provisions prohibiting unfair trade and competitive practices (especially in the instances of collaboration, merger or acquisition). The three pillars of U.S. antitrust law are the Sherman Act of 1890, the Clayton Act of 1914, and the FTC act of 1914. As many health systems move toward collaboration, combinations and closer relations, the presence of antitrust liability will have a definite impact on the future of health care delivery.

Appropriate and Necessary Health Services
Services needed to maintain an enrollee in good health including as a minimum, but not limited to, emergency care, inpatient hospital and physician care, outpatient health services and preventive health services delivered by authorized practitioners acting within their scope of practice.

Bad Debt Expense
Expenses from patient bills that the provider is unable to collect. Determination of bad debt expense usually is made after services are rendered and after debt collection efforts have failed.

Balanced Billing
Billing a patient for amounts over and above deductibles and copayments that are not reimbursed by the patient's insurance.

Benchmarking
The comparison of like physician's performance. A standard from which to establish what is "quality" medical care and develop measurement from which to evaluate providers and patient outcomes.

Beneficiary
A person who is eligible for or receiving benefits under an insurance policy or plan. The term is commonly applied to individuals receiving benefits through the Medicaid or Medicare programs or through a private health insurance plan.

Bundling
Combining into one payment the charges for various medical services rendered during one health care encounter. Bundling often combines the payment for physician and hospital services into one reimbursement. Also called "package pricing."

Canadian Health System
A form of the single payer model where the federal and provincial governments jointly handle the financing and administration of the health system. Financed mainly out of general tax revenues plus a payroll tax, the delivery system is composed of private doctors and hospitals, but each province establishes a fee schedule for physician payments and global budgets for hospitals. Built upon five principles—universality, accessibility, comprehensiveness, portability and public administration—Canada has crafted a unique health system for its citizens.

Capital Expenditure
An expenditure made for an asset with an expected useful life of more than one year.

Capitated Basis
A fixed per member per month payment or (less often) a percentage of premium paid to a provider who assumes the full risk of the cost of contracted services without regard to the type, value, or frequency of services provided.

Capitation
A method of reimbursement where organizations receive a fixed per member per month premium for each of their plan's covered lives. In return for this stream of revenue premiums, their plan provides a full range of health care services to its plan members. The organization bears the risk for the utilization of health care services and costs. An alternative to fee-for-service, this method is used primarily for HMO members but can be extended to EPO and POS plans. Although capitation payments can be based upon a number of criteria, such as the age and gender mix of the group, previous group experience, etc., the general structure is a flat rate *per member per month—or pm/pm.*

Physicians and/or hospitals can then be paid this amount each month for each member who has chosen that provider for services at open enrollment. This means that the enrollee selects a primary care physician (also known as a care coordinator or gatekeeper) and an associated hospital. The primary care physician is responsible for all services. Most plans allow the patient to change gatekeepers as often as once a month. These providers are then paid the flat rate for each member and are financially responsible for all services rendered regardless of the actual cost of providing the services. Capitation demands accurate recording and efficient procedures throughout the organization so that appropriate and medically necessary services are provided in an efficient and cost-effective manner. (See *Capitation Payment Systems*, page 57.)

Carve-outs

Risk adjustments made to capitated reimbursement arrangements to reallocate provider risk for services that the provider may not directly control, or which may pose an undesired financial risk (e.g., outpatient and inpatient facility charges).

Case Mix

A measure of the mix of cases being treated by a particular health care provider that reflects different levels of need for resources among different patient groups. Generally, case mix is established by estimating the relative frequency of the various types of patients seen by the provider involved during a given period and may be measured by factors such as diagnosis, severity of illness, utilization of services and provider characteristics.

Catchment Area

The geographic area from which a managed care organization draws its patients.

Charity Care

Health care services provided to individuals from whom the hospital or physician never expects to receive payment because of the patient's level of indigence. Thus, the charges incurred from the patients are written off to charity. It is sometimes very difficult to distinguish between charity care and bad debt expense.

Clinical Practice Guidelines

Systematically developed statements to assist provider and patient decisions about appropriate health care for specific clinical conditions.

Closed Panel

A managed care plan that contracts physicians on an exclusive basis. Physicians may be prohibited from seeing patients from other Managed Care Organizations (MCOs) (e.g., staff- and group-model HMOs).

Community Rating

Setting health insurance premiums based on the average costs of paying for services for all covered people in a geographical area, regardless of their individual history of (or potential for) using health services. Although this system was used successfully in the past, insurance companies generally do not set premiums based on community rating in today's environment. They try to relate premiums to the actual cost of services provided to each group of people they insure.

Continuous Quality Improvement (CQI)
A management system that emphasizes process management, customer service, waste reduction and people. In CQI, *continuous* means everyone participates and is integrated into all business functions in a never-ending process. *Quality* involves meeting or exceeding customer expectations. *Improvement* involves improving and maintaining business systems and their related processes.

Continuum of Care
A way of looking at the level and type of care provided to individuals from the most acute and intensive to the least acute and least intensive. The concept of the continuum is important because integrated health networks of the future will be expected to provide the entire range of services contained on the continuum.

Contractual Adjustments
That portion of a provider's charges or bills which is deemed noncollectible due to discount agreements with third-party payers. Payers use their leverage as volume buyers (number of plan enrollees) and their ability to route patients to specific providers to obtain contractual discounts.

Copayment
The portion of a specific claim or medical expense that an HMO member or insured person must pay out of pocket. This is usually a fixed amount and is justified as an incentive to discourage overuse of health services.

Cost Effective
A way of relating the cost of care to the achievement of a desired health outcome. The most cost-effective method is the one that achieves the health outcome at the least cost.

Cost Shifting
The practice of charging certain groups of patients higher rates to offset lower rates negotiated with, or mandated by, other payers.

Covered Service
This term refers to all of the medical services the enrollee may receive at no additional charge, or with an incidental copayment under the terms of the prepaid health care contract.

Direct Contracting
A negotiated arrangement between a hospital, a physician group and an employer where the provider agrees to offer price discounts (global pricing) for services to the employers. Typically, the employer agrees to limit its employees' ability to choose another provider. These plans usually cover services not related to workers' compensation claims.

Employer Buying Federation
An organization of companies formed to address a wide range of health care issues affecting employees of the individual companies. Many cities, such as Minneapolis, Cleveland and Miami, have seen their large employers band together to share information on hospital costs, service quality and clinical outcomes while also hoping to use their expanded size to negotiate better contracts with providers.

Encounter Level Data
Data related to the utilization of health care services by individual patients, enrollees or insureds, including claims data, abstracts of medical records and data from patient interviews and patient surveys.

Exclusive Provider Organization
This plan provides one level of benefits. Patients may only select from panel providers and there is no coverage for going out-of-network. Due to this restriction, EPO premiums can be priced to compete more closely with HMOs but maintain some of the freedom of choice of the PPO.

Experience Rating
A method of determining health plan premiums based on the historical utilization data and distinguishing characteristics of a specific subscriber group.

Explanation of Benefits (EOB)
A statement from the MCO detailing the service, the charge, the discount and the payment made for services delivered to an individual patient.

Federally Qualified HMO
A health maintenance organization (HMO) which has been determined by the U.S. Department of Health and Human Services (USDHHS) to meet the standards set forth in Title XIII of the Public Health Service Act, in such areas as financial and administrative stability, quality, scope of services covered, and rate-setting practices. An employer who provides health insurance coverage to employees may be required to offer a federally qualified HMO as an alternative to other health benefit plans offered.

Fee-for-Service
A traditional form of reimbursement in health care where payment is made based on services rendered to the patient. Whether payment is based upon usual, customary, and reasonable charges, allowable costs, or variations on these formats, health care providers are used to receiving reimbursement at some level for doing "things" (tests, procedures, etc.) for patients. With payers moving toward prospective pricing methods, such as DRGs and Capitation, providers are adjusting to bearing greater risk and responsibility for appropriate resource allocation and usage.

Fiscal Intermediary
A public or private organization that handles the processing and remittance of claims along with the reimbursement of providers for services. See Third Party Administrator.

501(c)3 Status
A category under the IRS statutes that classifies the guidelines for private, not-for-profit organizations. The statute stipulates that the organization classified as 501(c)3 must serve some public benefit and not allow for inurement (formal distribution of gains) to private individuals or groups. 501(c)3 qualifiers do not have to pay federal, state or local taxes on earnings. Not-for-profit does not mean that these organizations do not maintain a margin (excess revenues over expenses). Without a margin, there can be no investment to meet future growth and expansion needs.

Gatekeeper (Care Manager, Care Coordinator)
A *primary care* physician who is responsible (often financially and also clinically) for the care received by specific individuals in a managed care organization or other integrated health system. The primary care "gatekeeper" moves the person throughout the provider network, and patients cannot see a specialist physician without a referral from their primary care gatekeeper. The term gatekeeper has come under attack in the past few years and the terms care manager or care coordinator are becoming popular alternatives.

Group Practice Without Walls (GPWW)
A network of physicians who have merged into one legal entity but maintain each individual practice location. The assets of the individual practices have been acquired by a larger group, but some autonomy is retained at each site. Central management serves as the "owner" of both the facility and the equipment and also provides administrative services. If a network of independent physicians agrees to share certain administrative and managed care support services, this network could be called a *Clinic Without Walls*.

Group Purchaser
A person or organization purchasing health care services on behalf of an identified group of persons, regardless of whether the cost of coverage or services is paid for by the purchaser or by the persons receiving coverage or services. Group purchasers include, but are not limited to, health insurance plans offered by self-insured employers; group health coverage offered by fraternal organization, professional associations, or other organizations; state and federal health care programs; state and local public employee health plans; workers' compensation plans; and the medical component of automobile insurance coverage.

Guaranteed Issue
A component of insurance reform that requires insurers to cover applicants regardless of preexisting conditions, past claims medical history, claims experience and other factors.

Health Maintenance Organization (HMO)
An organization responsible for providing or arranging the provision of comprehensive health care services on a prepayment basis to voluntarily enrolled persons within a designated population. Some HMOs emphasize prevention, wellness and the "gatekeeper" model of primary care to maintain the health of their enrolled populations. Often the terms HMO and MCO are used interchangeably.

Health Outcome
A measure of the effectiveness of preventive or treatment health services, typically in terms of patient health status. Attributing changes in outcomes to health services requires distinguishing the effects of the many other factors that influence patients' health.

Health Promotion and Prevention
The process of fostering awareness, influencing attitudes and identifying alternatives so that individuals can make informed choices and change their behavior in order to achieve an optimum level of physical and mental health.

Health Status
The state of health of a specified individual, group, or population. Health status may be measured by obtaining people's subjective assessments of their health; by one or more indicators of mortality and morbidity in the population, such as longevity or maternal and

infant mortality; or by using the incidence or prevalence of major diseases. Most of these are of course, measures of disease status, but they are used as proxies in the absence of measures of either objective or subjective health. Conceptually, health status is the proper outcome measure for the effectiveness of a specific population's medical care system, although attempts to relate effects of available medical care to variations in health status have proved difficult.

Hold Harmless

The HMO may attempt to limit its liability by inserting a "hold harmless" clause in the physician's contract that shifts most or all of the liability onto the physician. The "hold harmless" provision says, in essence, that the physician agrees to hold the plan "harmless" for any liability that arises, or if anything bad or negative happens, the physician agrees to accept all responsibility for the care of the patient. Often there is the responsibility for the HMO or the physician to contract with secondary insurers to protect against catastrophic cases.

Hold Harmless and No Balance Billing Clauses

Most provider contracts contain a hold-harmless clause under which the provider agrees not to sue or assert any claims against the enrollee for services covered under the contract, even if the managed health care plan becomes insolvent or fails to meet its obligations.

A no-balance billing clause is similar (and may be used synonymously) and maintains that a provider may not balance bill a member for any payment owed by the plan, regardless of the reason for nonpayment. The provider may bill the member for any amount that member is required to pay, such as copayment or coinsurance, or for services not covered under the schedule of benefits (e.g., cosmetic surgery). Many state insurance departments (or other agencies having regulatory oversight in this area) will not approve the provider forms without inclusion of a hold-harmless clause with specific language. The Health Care Financing Administration (HCFA) also has adopted recommended model hold-harmless language applicable to federally qualified HMOs approved by the National Association of Insurance Commissioners.

A clause frequently found in managed care contracts, whereby the HMO and the physician hold each other to be not liable for malpractice or corporate malfeasance if either of the parties is found liable. This language does not preclude a managed care company from being sued if one of its physicians is sued. It may also refer to language that prohibits the provider from billing patients in the event a managed care company becomes insolvent. State and federal regulations may require this language.

Insured Services

Services that may be covered under the patient's HMO contract, but not as part of the capitated fee paid to the physician. The physician (medical group) may be able to bill the third party for additional prenegotiated fees for these services.

Integrated Delivery System (IDS)

(See *Integrated Delivery Systems (IDS)*, page 10.)

Independent Practice Association (IPA)

(See *Independent Practice Association (IPA)*, page 10.)

Integrated Provider Network (IPN)

A network created by physicians, hospitals and affiliated providers for purposes of sharing clinical and financial risk.

Long Term Care
Routine help with everyday activities such as eating, bathing and dressing necessitated because of chronic illness, disability or frailty. Long term care is provided to individuals in their homes, in community settings or nursing homes. A part of the continuum of care.

Managed Care/Managed Care Organizations (MCOs)
Managed care has been described in a variety of ways and you will see some other perspectives in this book as well. A basic definition would include:

> A form of health insurance coverage where enrollee utilization patterns and provider service patterns are monitored before (prospectively), during (concurrently), and after (retrospectively) the actual delivery of services. The insurer or other assigned intermediary engages in evaluations of providers to contain costs and ensue appropriate health service utilization by its members. Traditional indemnity insurance usually covered whatever the health care professional decided to do for the individual. However, managed care has the insurer playing a much more active role in determining what is done for a beneficiary, where it will be done, who will do it, and what they are willing to pay for it. Most businesses have determined managed care to be the best mechanism in controlling their health care costs. Managed care entities can be designated as *PPOs, HMOs, IPAs* or other alternative delivery systems.

Management Services Organization (MSO)
A business entity offering management and administrative services, such as practice management and billing, and contracting to providers through a direct contract, an affiliation arrangement, or indirectly through a subsidiary arrangement (sometimes a hospital subsidiary).

(See also page 11.)

Medicaid
The federal program created under Title XIX in the 1965 Amendments to the Social Security Act. It provides health care benefits to individuals categorically entitled to other federal welfare programs such as Aid to Families with Dependent Children (AFDC), Supplemental Security Income (SSI), and certain other groups (e.g., children and single mothers) who fall below the poverty level. This program is currently a strong topic in the budget reduction debates in Congress and is sure to undergo many changes very soon.

Medicare
A federal program created under Title XVIII of the 1965 Amendments to the Social Security Act. It primarily provides health insurance benefits to persons over the age of 65 and others eligible for Social Security Benefits.

Medicare, Part A
Part A is the Hospital Insurance Program of Medicare. It is the compulsory portion of Medicare that automatically enrolls (1) all persons aged 65 and over entitled to benefits under Old Age, Survivors, Disability and Health Insurance Program or railroad retirement; (2) persons under the age of 65 who have been eligible for disability for more than two years and; (3) insured workers (plus their dependents) requiring renal dialysis or kidney transplants.*

Medicare, Part B
Part B is the Supplemental Medical Insurance Program of Medicare. It is the voluntary portion of Medicare that includes coverage for physician services in which all persons entitled to Part A may enroll on a monthly premium basis.*

*This program is currently undergoing massive changes and the definitions provided here will soon be out of date.

Medicare Supplemental Plans
Medicare beneficiaries may be covered under an HMO in one of four ways.

1. If the Medicare beneficiary is still employed, he/she may be covered under the employer's HMO plan. A secondary portion of the beneficiary's services will be paid by Medicare.

2. Medicare beneficiaries may enroll in supplemental plans offered by an HMO. The patient pays the premium to the HMO for services not covered by Medicare.

3. Medicare patients also eligible for Medicaid may have their premiums for supplemental insurance paid by the state through Medicaid. (See *A Word About Medicare and Medicaid*, page 87.)

4. As of this writing, there is a great deal of legislation being discussed in the revamping of the Medicare program including patients being able to opt out of Medicare in favor of an HMO program.

Member Months
The number of prepaid patients enrolled in a given month. Member Months are used to determine the capitated amount.

Midlevel Practitioner (MLP)
Physicians' assistants, clinical nurse practitioners, nurse midwives, and the like; often called "associate providers." These are nonphysicians who deliver medical care, generally under the supervision of a physician, but at less cost.

Multi-hospital System
Two or more hospitals owned, leased, sponsored or contract managed by a central organization.

Outcomes Measurement
Recording the outcomes/results of health care intervention. Measuring outcomes allows comparison with the original situation of the patient and can test the treatment methods.

Outcomes Research
Research designed to identify and analyze the outcomes and costs of alternative interventions for a given clinical condition, in order to determine the most appropriate and cost-effective means to prevent, diagnose, treat or manage the condition. Outcomes research is also used to develop and test methods for reducing inappropriate or unnecessary variations in the type and frequency of interventions.

Peer Review Organization
An organization charged with reviewing quality and costs for Medicare. Generally operates at the state level.

Physician Hospital Organization (PHO)
An entity uniting a hospital (or hospital system) and a group of physicians (and possibly other providers) for the purpose of contracting with managed care plans.

(See also page 11.)

Practice Parameters
Strategies for patient management that are within the range of acceptable practices as established by professional organizations such as the medical specialty societies. Sometimes called *standards of practice,* practice parameters generally try to include all of the possible "accepted" ways of handling a particular patient. Other ways of describing defined patterns of care for particular cases/diagnoses include *clinical pathways, critical paths, standard treatment protocols, anticipated recovery paths and clinical progressions* to name a few.

Preexisting Condition
As defined by insurers, a condition existing before an insurance policy went into effect and commonly defined as one that would cause an ordinarily prudent person to seek diagnosis, care or treatment.

Preferred Provider Organization (PPO)
A plan or an organization that contracts with independent providers at a discounted fee for service. The providers may be governed by some type of utilization review. A PPO may be risk-bearing—such as an insurance company—or it may be non-risk-bearing—such as a physician-sponsored PPO that markets itself to insurance companies or self-insured companies. PPOs typically permit members to use non-PPO providers to higher levels of coinsurance or deductibles.

(See also page 11.)

Primary Care
Provision of basic or general health care by primary care physicians (most often family practitioners and general internists, though obstetrician/gynecologists and pediatricians are sometimes included), nurse practitioners, physician assistants, and other mid-level providers. Primary care often emphasizes those medical services required to maintain health or treat less complex and more common diseases. Patients usually enter the medical care system through primary care service providers.

Reinsurance
A type of insurance purchased by providers or MCOs to protect against specific risks. Reinsurance risk coverage may include individual stop-loss, aggregate stop-loss, out-of-area, and insolvency protection. As MCOs grow in membership, their reinsurance costs may be reduced by assuming such risks themselves and relying on larger reserves.

Repricer
A repricer is a third-party payer (i.e., an HMO) who pays the provider a flat annual amount per covered life, then charges the employer (or purchaser of the health care plan) for the cost of care plus a margin for profit. Cost of care is the per member per month dollar amount allocated for doctors, hospital care, and administrative expenses. Profit comes from the rate per member per month as sold to the employer less the cost. The role of the repricer is similar to a wholesaler or distributor providing the administrative cost to link the payer and the provider.

Resource Based Relative Value Scale (RBRVS)
The prospective payment system designed by the Health Care Financing Administration (HCFA) for Medicare physician reimbursement. It is currently the model on which some non-Medicare reimbursement systems are basing their payments. The components of this reimbursement mechanism are grouped around costs associated with the resources needed for overhead and skills/education. HCFA initially anticipated using RBRVS as a means of creating a more equitable payment balance between reimbursement for primary care physicians and specialists.

Risk Adjustment
A method of directing funds to MCOs with disproportionately sicker and/or harder to reach populations. Risk adjustments are designed to address the predictable variation in health plan costs related to the variance in age and health status in different enrollee populations.

Risk Withhold
This is the amount withheld from the physician's payment in a plan. This withheld amount is designed to cover plan costs that exceed an anticipated amount. If the plan is "cost effective," the physician may receive a refund of a portion of the amount withheld at the end of the plan year.

Shared Risk Services
Prepaid plans "budget" the dollar amount they anticipate paying for certain services such as inpatient hospital care, ambulance costs, inpatient hemodialysis, and extended care facility costs. If the amount they spend for these services is less than the budgeted amount, the physician or group may receive a share of these savings in additional payment. Conversely, if the actual costs for these services exceed the budgeted amount, the physician or group may be asked to pay into the fund part of the additional cost.

Stop-loss
In capitated arrangements for physicians, a form of reinsurance that provides protection for annual medical expenses above a certain limit. An example is protection for participating physicians for expenses over $2,500. When costs of a patient's care exceed that amount in a single year, the provider will be reimbursed for additional services at an agreed rate.

Third Party Administrator (TPA)
An entity that performs administrative functions (e.g., claims processing, membership enrollment, etc.) for a self-funded plan or a start-up managed care plan. A contracted independent organization that administers an employer's health plan. Most often TPAs process and pay claims, deal with benefit enrollment, etc.

(See also *Administrative Services Only.*)

Third Party Payer
Party to an insurance or prepayment agreement (usually an insurance company, prepayment plan or government agency) responsible for paying the provider designated expenses incurred on behalf of the insured.

Total Quality Management (TQM)
Systems and processes to identify and eliminate sources of error, waste, or redundancy by soliciting feedback and participation from all staff (especially non-management) and customers (i.e. patients). Also called continuous quality improvement (CQI).

(See also page 16.)

Triple Option Plan

These types of insurance plans typically contain three levels of benefits, each with various levels of flexibility to the insured. As flexibility increases, so does the amount the insured must pay out-of-pocket. These types of programs are also referred to as step-down benefit plans.

An example is an HMO allowing the insured to self-select a PPO-type plan or an indemnity plan at increased amounts of out-of-pocket expense to the insured. In doing so, the insured will have greater flexibility in the ability to choose a physician or a hospital and often will be less disrupted if an employer changes plans on an annual basis.

Utilization Management

A function of health services management that combines utilization review, risk management, and quality assurance in order to ensure prudent and effective use of provider resources and a high quality level of care. A strong internal utilization management program will have a positive influence on length of stay (create a decrease), resource utilization (ensure its appropriateness), labor force allocation (ensure proper level), and overall cost effectiveness of the organization.

Utilization Review

A formal assessment of the medical necessity, efficiency and/or appropriateness of health care services and treatment plans on a perspective, concurrent or retrospective basis.

Value

The desired clinical outcome and level of service at an acceptable price to the purchaser and consumer of health care services.

CHAPTER 2

Physician Roles in Managed Care

The Role of the Primary Care Physician ("Gatekeeper")

What is the role today of primary care physicians in a managed health care system? The primary care provider controls primary patient access to services that include comprehensive care, coordinated care and a continuum of care.

Who delivers on these commitments? Generally, family practitioners and general internists are considered primary care physicians. In some regions, obstetrician-gynecologists and pediatricians have also been designated as primary care providers or serve in a collaborative role with the family practitioner and internist. The primary care physician is the patient's personal physician and acts as the patient's advocate. This physician is the medical professional to whom the patient must often turn for care, overall guidance and ongoing support in the context of a long-term physician-patient relationship.

In most well-run managed care systems, an adult primary care physician will have a designated panel of 3,000 to 4,000 patients, depending on the age and illness mix of the population (a 100 percent Medicare panel would have 700–1,000 patients). The primary care physician serves as the main point of health care access. Most health care comes through this physician though there are often exceptions in the areas of mental health, obstetrical services and dermatology. Some systems allow referral to a second specialist once an initial specialist has been seen.

This access coordination feature of managed care plans is criticized sometimes by specialists. However, it is essential in assisting the primary care physicians in following their patients and coordinating care. Primary care physicians will "keep track" of their patients through phone calls, written consultative reports from the specialist, hospital visits and the like. The skilled primary care physician will work with the specialists to develop a collegial, as opposed to competitive, relationship based upon delivering the most appropriate care to the patient.

Continuity of care is the third aspect of the role of the primary care physician. The primary physician must be available to the patient on an ongoing basis to ensure effective coordination. This is particularly true for adults with complex and chronic conditions. It may be less problematic for healthy children and young adults. Even with good recordkeeping and automated medical records, care will be more efficient and problems more quickly sorted out if the physician is familiar with the patient.

The fourth aspect of the primary care physician's role relates to the comprehensive provision of services. The physician is responsible for seeing that comprehensive services are provided and is accountable, at least in part, for all care that is rendered to the patient. This ranges from basic preventive services to care in the intensive care unit. This might include direct care or collaborative care for patients with diabetes, rheumatoid arthritis, and HIV who might have seen only specialists in a nonmanaged system. The role of the primary care physician is critical. Computerized reminder systems now enhance the ability of many primary care physicians to perform preventive tasks and improve care. Some primary care physicians in managed care plans shy away from assuming such a broad and central role in the patient's care. By doing so, they make the jobs of their specialist colleagues and everyone else involved more difficult and less efficient.

The role of the primary care physician in a managed health care system is most completely described by the term *personal care manager*. This concept combines all the previous noted attributes—those of a personal primary care physician — with those of an effective case manager. A case manager is a coordinator of care, a "manager of the system" for the patient. The case management process is one of matching the patients' needs and preferences with the judicious use of medical services. There are five key roles for the primary care physician case manager—*navigator, negotiator, evaluator, educator, and decision maker.*

- **Navigator**
  The navigator assumes the role of helping the patient move through the system, smoothly and efficiently, with minimal emotional and financial trauma. His responsibility is to chart the course, measure and manage the outcomes.

- **Negotiator**
  The negotiator works directly with the patient, physician colleagues, support personnel, and other professionals to determine a course of treatment and an action plan for the patient's care. Effective case management relates to the ability to negotiate and communicate clearly with coworkers. Negotiating with patients is also sometimes necessary.

- **Evaluator**
  The evaluator provides critical evaluation and assessment of various treatment modalities, even those provided by another physician. Specialized knowledge is critically important in the care of patients. Equally important is the ability to critically evaluate information, ask the right questions, compare alternatives, and know when information is incomplete. The effective primary care case manager asks the tough but obvious questions. Because the primary care physician is trained in medical decision making and clinical epidemiology, clinical problem solving may be approached more scientifically.

- **Educator**
  This role relates to the willingness and ability to communicate with patients regarding their medical problems and how they can be managed conservatively, how to access and use the health care system, and what to expect with care and services. It means taking the time to explain, in a caring and scientific way, that back sprains rarely require a CT scan or even an X-ray, that overprescribing antibiotics for upper respiratory infections may result in resistant strains of bacteria, that most headaches are not evaluated best with an MRI scan, and that a sensation of a skipped heartbeat does not mean that one must see a cardiologist. Most patients are reassured if the physician is confident, caring and has demonstrated good judgment in the past.

  The educator role applies to preventive health services and includes teaching patients how frequently services are needed, which services are actually useful for screening, and how to take care of one's self when under the supervision of a physician. Midlevel practitioners (physician assistants, associate providers, and nurse practitioners) can be particularly effective in performing these tasks and other basic primary care functions.

- **Decision Maker**
  The decision maker role brings together all the physician's skills, knowledge of the patient, personal experience, trending data, and in some situations clinical algorithms, to enable the physician to make a clinical decision with the patient. The probabilities of a certain clinical outcome are weighed against the risks and costs of testing or treating.

Qualities and Capabilities of a Personal Care Manager

The highly capable primary care physician who can act as a personal care manager has skills and competencies in three basic areas. They are:

- Organization and practice management skills, such as
  - familiarity with quality improvement and utilization management
  - understanding of ethical and legal considerations
  - team building
  - design and oversight of office systems
  - financial management issues
  - cost effectiveness

- Personal characteristics such as attitudes toward patients, professional teams, and individual colleagues are demonstrated by the following traits:
  - respects and listens to others' opinions
  - tolerates and manages conflict
  - serves in a facilitating and problem solving role

- Clinical skills, such as:
  - supports and provides preventive care

Management Tools

Following are some common tools used by the primary care physician in a managed care system to provide high-quality, cost-effective care:

- Hospital Utilization Rates — generally used to assess the performance of entire groups of physicians and patients.

- Referral Rates — used to compare among same-specialty physicians the types of conditions for which patients are referred.

- Pharmacy Use Rates, Costs, Drug Interactions — the number of prescriptions per member per year, used to assess the performance of the entire group.

- Laboratory Use Rates, Costs — used to assess the number of tests per encounter, laboratory costs per encounter, total laboratory costs, the types of tests ordered.

- Imaging Use Rate, Costs — used to asses total imaging costs per physician per encounter, or per month.

- Procedure Use Rates — numerous procedures are now trended, usually expressed in terms of the number per 1,000 members per year.

- Preventive Service Rates — the rates at which certain preventive services are provided to the entire covered population, these can be assessed at the group level, and with a good information system, also at the individual level.

- Hospital Readmission Rates, Surgical Complication Rates — statistics that provide some indication of the quality of hospital care.

- Member Satisfaction Rates — conducted to gain feedback and trending information for individual physicians, surveys often include specific areas that cause, or detract from satisfaction among patients with their physicians.

- Automated Patient Tracking/Reminder Systems and Computerized Patient Records — to assist physicians in their ongoing management of patients, these systems are useful because they help physicians retrieve readily available information that is important to good clinical care.

- Clinical Algorithms/Protocols and Practice Guidelines — these serve as templates for decision making with respect to many common clinical problems, in both the inpatient and outpatient settings. Computerized information systems can be used to quickly retrieve data to measure physician performance, individually and collectively, against these guidelines.

The Role of the Nonprimary Care Physician Specialist

What is the role of the nonprimary care specialist physician in most managed care systems? The answer depends on the patient, the situation, the physician involved, the plan design, and the local community practice. The specialist physician's role for a given patient is linked to the type of illness or condition that the patient has, and to the severity of the illness or condition. Once the primary physician assesses the body system involved, the possible disease state, and the potential severity of the condition, the specialist physician may become involved.

The specialist physician's role may take the form of that of a consultant, an expert diagnostician, or an acute rehabilitator, depending on whether the patient has an acute or chronic illness and condition.

- **Consultant** — a consultant's role is clearly a supportive role. It involves making an assessment and a recommendation based on information conveyed directly from the primary care physician, or the physician and the patient. The primary physician performs a workup and poses a focused set of questions to the consultant.

- **Expert Diagnostician** — not all patients can be completely evaluated by the primary care physician, nor can all patients who are referred to specialists be properly assessed with a single visit and one or two simple diagnostic tests. Some patients require intensive evaluation and a significant diagnostic procedure. For these, and many more, the specialist plays a critical role in using modern technology to determine the source of the problem, or whether there is a problem. Once a diagnosis is made the specialist also plays an important role in either formulating a therapeutic plan or assisting the primary care physician in developing and implementing the plan.

- **Acute Rehabilitator** — the specialist takes on this role when the patient has an acute illness or condition and the primary physician determines that the specialist needs to see the patient immediately. It is very important that the primary care physician recognize the condition early and involve the specialist as soon as possible. The primary care physician should continue to be involved directly in the patient's care to observe the flow of events, facilitate communication among specialists, keep the patient and family fully informed, and generally coordinate the activities by working closely with the principal specialist.

For chronic illnesses and conditions, the specialist has two roles. The first role is to be a consultant. The specialist's advice is very useful when, over time, the patient with a chronic illness experiences changes that suggest an increasing severity of the condition or the possible need for change in medication or therapy. Second, as a periodic reviewer of care for a patient with a chronic illness, usually a more serious one. Depending on the diagnosis, the schedule may vary from as few as one or two visits over several months to several visits over several years. The follow-up schedule should be spelled out clearly and followed scrupulously.

The specialist has a very important role to play as an educator in both acute and chronic illness. He serves in a collaborative role with primary care physicians in these cases. Patient education is not provided solely in the primary care physician's office. Patients with complex illnesses or medical problems that require a specialist may have intensive educational needs that the specialist is best prepared to address. The specialist with extensive clinical experience in a particular discipline, is best able to communicate to the patient a prognosis or the natural course of the illness.

Specialists can also play an important role in educating their primary care physician colleagues about the particulars and nuances of certain clinical conditions and the types of patients who need referrals. One effective way is through clinical conferences.

Qualities and Capabilities of a Specialist

The specialist in any discipline needs to be:

- well trained
- dedicated to timely communication
- able to provide a critical analysis of information
- a judicious user of resources

Additionally, it is important to have the following attitudes:

- demonstrate a willingness to collaborate and communicate
- be open to learning how to perform in a new and more efficient manner
- have a clear understanding on how responsibilities are executed in conjunction with primary care physicians

In this way, the specialist can have a positive influence on supporting quality, cost-effective care for the patient.

Management Tools

In addition to the tools described for primary care physicians, specialist physicians may obtain ad hoc reports that allow them to evaluate the total cost per case for a procedure, or for a period of illness. For example,

- Cost profiles — may contain hospital-based services that are not part of the direct bill of the specialist, but they are services that the specialist can influence. In this way, the specialist can have impact on the cost and quality of hospital care.

- Trending reports — allow the evaluation of entire populations of individuals with certain medical problems. These types of data are usually of great interest to physicians and allow them to better understand the types of patients they are seeing and what happens to them over time.

To summarize, mostly the use of "specialists" means nonprimary care physician specialists. All serious participants recognize primary care physicians as specialists. The roles described provide a general overview of how the primary care physician and the specialist physician operate in many MCOs. This does not imply that all primary care physicians accept these broad roles. However, as involvement in managed care increases, primary care training programs are emerging to enhance physicians' skills.

It is very important that physicians play strong leadership roles in managed health care systems. Physicians are in the best position to understand the needs and desires of patients and to respond to them. It is critical that there is a strong, positive working relationship between primary care and nonprimary care specialists. This requires extensive communication, organized planning, sharing of information at the doctor-to-doctor level, the group or specialty department level and the doctor-to-MCO level. Physicians need to meet regularly to discuss how certain clinical problems will be managed. They need to develop protocols and guidelines and examine and manage costs. Their activities need to be facilitated by an effective clinical leader, and they must be driven by credible data. Good organization and good leadership are critically important.

Information will become increasingly important for managing the care process. The ability to retrieve, analyze, and disseminate information rapidly and effectively lies at the heart of the managed care system.

These are exciting times in health care with great possibilities for markedly improving the health care system. Despite the understandable fears and concerns of many physicians today, there are reasons to be optimistic that physicians will adapt to the changes that are associated with managed health care and make it a far better approach to care than it has ever been before.

CHAPTER 3

Developing a Managed Care Strategy

A fundamental business relationship in managed care is the direct contract between the physician and insurance company or MCO. This is a dramatic departure from the traditional roles in the physician/patient business relationship. In the past, the patient has been responsible for payment beyond those made by their insurance plans. Patients and providers, however, have traditionally been "protected" from looking at costs — especially patients who have enjoyed first dollar coverage plans. Today, insurance companies with sophisticated negotiating and contracting expertise are seeking formal business relationships with physicians. Therefore, *it is imperative that physicians develop a strategy to evaluate both new and existing contracts from insurance companies and MCOs.*

To develop an effective strategy, you must go through the following steps:

- **Assessing your practice**
    - Financial information

        Note: In gathering and analyzing this data, be sure you look at the difference between the charges for providing care and the cost of providing that care in your practice setting.

    - Practice geographic and demographic information
    - Practice capacity and capability
    - Referral sources
    - Management information systems
    - Competition
    - Cost effectiveness and efficiency
    - Patient satisfaction

- **Assessing proposed contracts**
    - Obtain information on the managed care organization
    - Obtain information about the plan
    - Obtain references from current participants
        - Detailed review of the contract
        - Obligations of the managed care plan
        - Obligations of the physician
    - Impact of system participation on practice
    - Plan payment methodology

Chapter 3 — Developing a Managed Care Strategy   31

- Utilization review and quality assurance provisions
- Appeal process
- Term and termination

■ **Assessing the effectiveness of existing contracts**
- (See Chapter 8 for assessing payment effectiveness of a managed care plan)
- Number of patients covered by plan
- Revenue, adjustments (discounts), costs by patient
- Comparison with other existing plans

Assessing the Current Practice

To begin developing a managed care strategy, evaluate the practice from two perspectives: First, your own professional well-being and goals; secondly, from the viewpoint of the payer, the managed care organization, and patient. Look at the practice as a business — one that sells services. This premise represents a swing away from the traditional physician's core identity as a professional providing a range of services.

Take a thorough look at the practice by gathering the following information:

Financial Information
Compile the following information from the past three years. (Maintain the information for future trend analyses.)

■ Explanation of Benefits (EOBs) from all payers
- Charges per month
- Payment per month
- Adjustments per month

■ Outstanding accounts receivable each month for each payer

■ Practice overhead costs by month
- Staffing costs
- Rent/lease
- Medical supplies

Practice Geographic and Demographic Information
Compile the following information from the past three years. (Without an advanced tracking system, this information is not readily attained. This data should be maintained for future trend analysis.)

■ Procedures by code and payer each month

■ New patients by payer each month

■ Referrals by payer each month

■ Hospital admissions by payer each month

■ Patient turnover — how many calls do you get for records transfer and why?

- Staff turnover—this is an expensive item in most practices. If the staff is turning over, determine why and make adjustments as possible.

Practice Capacity and Capabilities

- Determine the number of new patients the practice can accept without adding staff.
- Review the average wait for a new patient to get an appointment (10 weeks).
- Review the average waiting time for appointment to be seen (1 hour).
- Determine hardships imposed if practice office hours were changed.
- Determine competitive risks if practice office hours are not changed.

Assessing Proposed Contracts

After looking at the practice and drawing conclusions about its strengths and weaknesses, it is time to evaluate the managed care organization's market area. In addition, the MCO must be financially sound and of good reputation. Obtain the following information about the plan.

General Plan Information

- List of physicians in your geographic area who currently participate in the plan. (Focus on physicians in your specialty and those to whom you currently refer patients. Also try to obtain information regarding physicians who have been eliminated from the plan in the past 12-18 months—either through their decision or the plan's—and the reasons why.)
- Market share and program growth history of the plan
- Compliance or complaints registered with state regulatory agency
- Ownership of the managed care organization and their most recent annual report

Financial Information

- Capitated Plan
  - Projected number of subscribers
  - Reimbursement
  - Potential ability for MCO to change patient base
- Discounted Fee-for-service Plan
  - Basis for fee schedule, (e.g., McGraw-Hill or RVS)
  - Obtain plan's payment rates for procedures you do most often
  - Provide a listing of your top twenty revenue generating procedures/services, without the prices, to the managed care organization for comparison

Employer/Employee Information

- Number of new employers signed within the last year
- Complete list of employers in the area that offer the plan
- Percentage of penetration (among employees) the plan has enrolled in the plan
- Number of employees in the plan living in your patient catchment area
- Average age of participants in the plan

Obtain References From Current Participants

- Contact the offices of several physicians who participate in the plan(s) you are considering. Ask the practice manager or reimbursement specialist in that practice the following questions:
    - If this is a fee-for-service plan, what is the turn-around time for payment of a submitted bill? If it is a capitated plan, do payments arrive as promised?
    - Does an updated list of current enrollees accompany the capitation check each month?
    - How many claim denials do they average each month?
    - What are the specific administrative or procedural problems?
    - What is the average age of their accounts receivable in the plan?
    - If the plan is a discounted fee-for-service, what percentage of their full fee does it cover?
    - Has participation in the plan increased the patient base and **added** revenue to the practice?
    - When the plan's premiums increase, have you seen a corresponding adjustment in your reimbursement?

Managed Care Contract Review Steps

To review managed care contracts, begin with a four-step system:

Step 1: Gather Information. Begin by gathering the following documents.

- Complete copy of the contract
- Provider handbook (office manual or administrative guide)
- Full fee schedule (physician's and plan's)
- Complete list of covered services (specialty specific).
- Patient contract with MCO
- Detailed procedure for eligibility/coverage verification
- Complete Utilization Review protocol/procedures
- Complete Quality Assurance protocol/procedures
- Detailed dispute resolution protocol/procedures
- Provider listing
- Marketing materials
- Other

Step 2. Perform Financial Screen or Analysis. Here is how.

- List your most financially significant or frequently used CPT codes (or all, if possible); multiply your standard fees by the annual frequency for each code to *determine your standard earnings.* Then for each code, multiply the (net) plan fee times the annual frequency to *determine the plan earnings.* (See table to the right.)

- Determine overhead expenses, which are your annual total expenses excluding physician compensation.

- Compare plan earnings and overhead expenses. If earnings are greater than expenses, you can conclude the MCO reimburses enough to make some contribution to physician compensation.

- Compare physician compensation under standard earnings with that under plan earnings. Physician compensation is what is left over from each earnings calculation after subtracting overhead expenses. Determine the percentage reduction in physician compensation. Is this percentage acceptable?

CPT Code	Standard Fee	Annual Frequency	Standard Earnings	Plan Fee (Net)	Annual Frequency	Plan Earnings
11200	45	6	270	30	6	180
14001	110	4	440	108	4	432
56303	1350	18	24300	750	18	13500
58100	1485	33	49005	783	33	25839
58410	1275	12	15300	688	12	8256
59430	650	25	16250	325	25	8125
76815	125	129	16125	96	129	12384
81002	12	456	5472	7	456	3192
84144	25	54	1350	12	54	648
85014	25	658	16450	16	658	10528
85025	22	126	2772	11	126	1386
99203	57	982	55974	51	982	50082
99212	54	325	17550	49	325	15925
99213	63	837	52731	56	837	46872
Total			**$273,989**			**$197,349**

Assume this is ALL of the work you did in a year and that your total expenses EXCLUDING physician compensation for the year are $142,000.

Step 3. Perform Background Check/Review Terms and Conditions. The following checklist provides a starting point for a critical review of a proposed contract. By answering the following questions, you will focus on the effect of a proposed contract on your medical practice; on the need to obtain and review other documents from the MCO; and on topics to discuss with office personnel and other physicians who have experience with a particular MCO.

Assessing the Managed Care Organization

- Who is the owner?

- What is the MCO's market share?

- How many covered lives? How much has it grown over the last six months, i.e., covered lives *added*?

- What are target markets and prospects for the future?

- What physicians, hospitals, pharmacies, and ancillary services contract with the managed care organization and are available to serve your patients? Do you have preexisting relationships with them? What drugs are included on the formulary?

- Who is on the Board of Directors?

- Who is the Medical Director?

- What is the financial status? Is it profitable? Are premiums stable? Are withholds returned?

- What accreditation does it have? NCQA? Dunn & Bradstreet? Moodys? Other?

- Is it licensed by state bureaus? What states? Does the bureau have a list of complaints or malpractice suits brought against it?

Review Financial Terms

- Obtain a complete and specialty specific fee schedule. Determine what is not covered. If this is impossible to obtain, provide the MCO a list of your 20 most financially significant or frequently provided services with CPT codes and your fees. Ask specifically if these services are covered by the plan and what is the fee paid.

- Ask about withholds, risk pools. How and when is repayment made? What is the auditability of withholds and risk pools? Is the physician liable for increased pay back if the plan's budget is not met?

- Timing of payments, billing limits. When does the MCO promise payment? Do they pay on time? Do they often question valid submitted claims?

Review Terms and Conditions

- What services are covered?

- What is the authorization process? What are the requirements for prior authorization, and is the mechanism reasonably available when needed? What preauthorization or other requirements are established for referring to a specialty physician, nonphysician provider, or facility?

- What are the benefit limitations/exclusions?

- What is the process for verifying enrollment and eligibility status?

- What are the levels of malpractice coverage required of the physician? Does the MCO have malpractice coverage and what are the limits?

- What are the levels of financial liability for the physician? For the MCO? What are your obligations if the plan goes bankrupt or becomes insolvent? Does the plan have insolvency insurance?

- What are the obligations for providing covered services (i.e., schedule, location)? Does the contract require you to be available on a 24-hour basis? What are the requirements for on-call coverage, emergency appointments, and patient access?

- Must you accept all patients referred to you? Are there maximum or minimum numbers of enrollees you must accept?

- If you close your practice to new patients enrolled in that plan, are you restricted to close your practice to other plans or patients?

- What is the full scope of responsibilities of primary care physicians? Can patients self-refer to subspecialists?

Review General Clauses

- If a plan is a PPO (or PHO), will the physician automatically become a part of any new benefit plan the PPO accepts, without notice? If so, how will the physician be notified? Will he be dropped from the entire plan if he refuses to participate in a new benefit plan? Will his entire contract with the plan be terminated? Will the fee schedule for any new benefit plan accepted by the PPO be the same as the fee schedule provided in the original contract signed by the physician?

- Is there a clause to prohibit the assignment of benefits or delegation of obligations without prior written consent of both parties? *Assignment to another entity can result in the contracting physician doing business with an entity other than the one evaluated and selected.*

- Does the contract obligate you to perform any services after the contract is terminated? What are the time limits or parameters for delivery of services?

- How are disputes resolved between the physician and the MCO? By arbitration or by legal process? Who bears the expense?

- Who has final authority for patient care?

- Are there provisions in the contract that incorporate amendments "by reference?" If the contract states that the physician will be required to comply with all policies, procedures and standards enacted by amendment by the MCO or payer, do you have the opportunity both to review and maintain copies of such documents? Will you be advised of modifications to these documents? Are you bound by any modifications?

- Does the contract say that a written amendment is the only way to amend the document?

- Can the contract be terminated with or without cause by either party? What are the specific "causes" which would constitute a breach of contract and lead to termination?

- Who is responsible for notifying patients in the event of termination? Who is responsible for copying the medical records of enrollees if the contract is terminated? Who bears the expense?

- Does the contract prohibit you from taking any action or making any communication that undermines or could undermine the confidence of patients, potential patients, their employers, their unions, or the public in the MCO, or the quality of care that it provides?

- Does the contract "hold harmless" enrollees from any responsibility for bills for services covered by the prepaid plan, even if the patient's bills are not paid by the MCO (for any reason, including insolvency or failure to make timely payment by the organization)?

- Must you indemnify the MCO against liability? If so, does your professional liability policy cover this? *Consult with your malpractice carrier for advice. If your policy does not cover this, such a provision could obligate you to a potentially large exposure.*

- Is there a provision addressing what happens when treatment is wrongfully denied or harmful delays are caused due to preauthorization mechanisms of the MCO? What happens if these events occur?

- Is the process of appealing a peer review decision reasonable and acceptable? Are limitations on referrals realistic? When are they required, and are they readily available?

- Is the physician required to participate in peer review? Does the plan protect the physician from liability?

Step 4. Making the Decision to Participate. Certain provisions of a contract may either make or break your decision to sign a proposed contract. Following are areas of further opportunity or future problems.

- **Deal Killers.** When reviewing a contract, be particularly watchful for any of the following clauses. Any one of these provisions may be reason enough to avoid signing an agreement.

    - Reimbursement will be less than your overhead costs for providing services.

    - The percentage reduction in physician compensation is greater than an acceptable limit.

    - The contract requires the assumption by the practice of obligations of the MCO (i.e., the physician and MCO are not clearly independent parties). The contract should confirm the relationship of the MCO and the physician as independent entities contracting with each other solely to effect the provision of the Agreement.

    - The contract contains a "hold harmless" clause that is for the physician only.

    - The contract terms are alterable at the will of the MCO (they can make unilateral amendments) without prior notice to you and/or without your prior consent. *The physician should have 30 days written notice of any changes or amendments to the contract.*

    - The contract has no provisions for appealing adverse Utilization Review, Quality Assurance, and Medical Management Decisions.

- **Tie Breakers.** Guard against any of the other stipulations in an agreement that may not work in the best interest of your practice. Give careful consideration before signing a contract with these provisions:

    - Billing limits under 90 days. *The contracting physicians should review billing requirements. Seek a sixty-day period that begins with the end of the month in which service is rendered.*

    - Exclusivity. *No language should be included in the agreement that restricts the physician from entering into other contracts or agreements to provide health care services to other health care plans, insurers, patients or employer groups. Neither should the MCO be restricted from entering into contracts nor agreements with other physicians or parties.*

    - Ability to assign without notice/approval. *This clause is not recommended.*

    - Ability to retroactively deny payment.

- Payment period beyond 45 days. It is crucial that a managed care agreement has a definite due date for payments. *In general, a due date of 30 days is prompt and fair.*
- Presence of "gag clause" which prohibits you from taking any action or making any communication about the quality of care the MCO provides.

Once you have completed your four-step review, you are prepared to make a decision about your contractual relationship with an MCO. With your strategic plan in hand, and your written summary results or conclusions drawn from (1) financial indicators, (2) MCO assessment, (3) operational impact, and (4) legal assessment, you are ready to negotiate, sign or decline the agreement.

CHAPTER 4

Assessing the Impact on Your Practice

Before signing a contract to participate in a plan, an important step to take is assessing the impact on the practice. The following issues should be considered regarding practice capacity, patient source, and costs.

Practice Capacity

The physician or group must look at the practice to determine whether there is capacity to accept new patients. Consideration of the following can help with this determination.

- *What is the average number of patients seen in the office per week?*

    Consider the number of patients you would likely receive from the MCO.

    - Could your practice absorb those patients with the current staff? If not, how available is more staff and what would you need to add?

    - Would you need to extend your office hours or days the practice is open to include longer hours during the week and on weekends? How accommodating would your physician and support staff be to this potential change?

    - What are the retirement plans of your colleagues? Will you need to add physicians and/or mid-level practitioners in the future? What is the market in your area regarding physician supply?

    - How long does it take on average to recruit a new physician and at what cost? (Often the recruitment specialists at the local hospital can supply this information. Ask for information on starting salaries, signing bonuses, relocation expenses, etc.) Would you need to hire an outside recruiter for this task and at what price?

    - The questions regarding physician supply and demand should be periodically reviewed by a practice regardless of consideration of an MCO. Primary care physicians especially can be difficult to recruit.

- *What is the average number of hospital visits or consults per week?*

    As in the discussion above, this information will feed your analysis of how you might need to staff for absorption of a patient population from an MCO contract.

    - Consider the patient demographics available to you from the MCO to estimate this variable.

    - If your practice already has a considerable hospital practice, it may not be difficult to add a few more patients to an existing load.

    - If you are primarily clinic-based, however, consideration should be given to this issue including the impact hospital coverage may have on your call schedule.

- *How long must new patients wait for an available appointment?*

    Waiting times for appointments may need to be contractually agreed to depending upon the MCO contract.

    - In looking at this issue, consider your current patient population as well as the potential new patient base. Also look to see if all physicians in your group have approximately the same amount of waiting time. If they do not, check to see how the schedule may be more evenly spread. Review patient satisfaction surveys to see if patients do not make return appointments with a particular physician in the group and if not, why not.

    - Also consider what types of patients mid-level practitioners in your practice are or could be seeing. This is a useful, annual exercise to evaluate the productivity of individuals and their support staff in the overall contribution to the group regardless of an MCO affiliation.

If you have capacity to add new patients with a minimal increase in overhead, you should seriously consider doing so. Though you usually will be receiving a discounted fee, you may not see a measurable offset in expenses, making this potentially a wise financial decision. If you will need to add staff or space to accommodate a new patient population, carefully consider this option against the length of the contract, the number of patient visits over what period of time it would take to break even, and similar considerations.

Patient Source Analysis

It is surprising how many independent practices do not have a firm understanding of the source of their patients. To anticipate future moves within the local market, perform an analysis on a quarterly basis. Below are some areas to consider in this review:

- *How many patients are referred to your practice each year?*

    Logging and utilizing the information on new patients is very important when considering current and future staffing needs of your practice and looking at long-term practice capacity. In addition to discerning the number of patients, find out where they came from.

    - Did you participate in a marketing campaign that yielded strong results?

    - Did your practice speak at an event or staff a health screening?

    - Are you giving wellness classes or serving as the team doctor for the local high school? Are referrals coming from there? As the demand for your time increases, consider the net patient referral when you are assigning priorities to "outside" activities.

- *What physicians referred patients to you?*

    Look at the top five or so physicians who referred patients to your practice and consider the following:

    - Did their associates also refer?

    - What types of patients did they send to you?

    - What is your relationship to that physician? Is it one-way or reciprocal?

    - To which managed care plans do these physicians belong?

- *Who are the large employers in your market area?*

    Analyzing your patient population according to their employees is important especially if there are one or two larger employers in the area that make up most of the population or most of the patient base of your practice. If any of these companies are heavily represented in your practice, think about what the impact would be if they joined a managed care plan in which you did not participate. The local hospital administration may have an idea of what the larger employers in the area are considering and can keep you abreast of what their future plans might be. Often, especially in smaller communities, you may have enough social capital to access this information.

Never underestimate the costs to these employers of providing health care benefits for their work force. In this competitive era, they will surely be looking at these costs often to determine if there are ways to reduce their overhead. Managed care plans are eager to help them with this process.

By participating in an analysis of your patient sources, you are in a better position to consider your options. Request that your colleagues notify you if they are considering participation with a new plan. You can then consider the impact this will have on your referrals.

Service Analysis

- *What services and/or procedures are required of the physician under the proposed managed care plan?*

    Often the MCO will require the primary care physician to perform certain procedures or services. If you are equipped to offer these services in your office and they are part of your current overhead, there are minimal new costs involved. However, if you must purchase new equipment and aquire staff and/or training, consider those overhead expenses in your analysis. Look at not only the equipment, but also the time commitments that will affect your ability to schedule patients in your current appointment work flow.

- *If capitated, what ancillary services are included in the capitation rate?*

    Especially if you refer ancillary procedures to another physician or vendor, consider the cost structure of providing these services. This consideration should include what contractual arrangements are in place (for example, referral to an outside laboratory) and the costs of bringing those services into your office.

- *Who pays for services and/or procedures referred out of the practice?*

    If you are responsible for payment in your per member per month rate, consider not only the cost and frequency of these services, but whether or not the MCO restricts your choice of vendors. If so, at what cost?

Cost Analysis

Once you have gathered the data, you can better determine your cost to provide service. One way to organize this data is to produce a grid that resembles the one below.

Top Ten Procedures	Professional Charges	Ancillary Charges	Average Revenue per Patient Visit	Total Fixed Expenses per Year	Total Variable Expenses per Year	Average Expense per Patient Visit	MCO Revenue per Patient Visit

The *top ten procedures* for your practice should encompass approximately 80 percent of your patient base. If it does not, you may want to take the analysis deeper.

Professional fees should not include ancillary, injection or other similar charges.

Ancillary charges are broken away from professional fees so one can consider them separately, depending upon the terms of any managed care plan. This also helps in the negotiation of fees if you utilize an outside laboratory or other services.

Total fixed expenses per year must include space rental and leasehold improvements, amortization of capital expenses, insurance (malpractice and building) and utilities. Other fixed expenses are association dues for the practice, accounting fees and the like.

Total variable expenses should include staffing expense (including physician salaries) and other expenses that vary based upon the volume of patient visits.

Average expense per patient visit yields the expense you will want to compare to the revenue being offered by the MCO. From that information, you can quickly estimate the volume of patients you must see to cover your expenses and maintain your income stream.

Other considerations should include the number of days in accounts receivable and the anticipated receivable days of the MCO, from billing to date of payment. This will help you estimate whether you would encounter any cash flow issues.

Once you have set up this system with actual data from your practice, you are in a better position to evaluate your current status. You can weigh the impact of continuing unchanged or participating in one or more managed care plans.

All of the cost data should be considered along with the information you have gathered regarding your practice capacity, patient sources and required services. The competitive environment in your area is equally important to your analysis and necessary for building a complete picture for basing these important decisions.

This analysis should be ongoing. In our current health care environment, many outside forces will affect you and your practice. Review this data often (quarterly is preferable) so you can anticipate changes you may wish to make to assure your long-term financial viability.

CHAPTER 5

Payment Effectiveness of a Managed Care Contract

The managed care environment has created a need for the physician's office to track, analyze and develop strategies in managing their managed care plans. The following steps provide the foundation for building an effective managed care tracking system. Setting up this system will ensure that the practice performs ongoing evaluation and improvement of its managed care strategy.

Steps:

1. Determine the number of patients in the practice covered by each plan.

2. Determine the revenue generated by each plan.

3. Determine the adjustments (discount rate) made necessary by participating with each plan.

4. Compare this information with all other payers.

5. Analyze the net revenue per patient and the profit columns to determine which plans contribute the strongest revenue streams.

The following graph represents six managed care plans with varying amounts of revenue, costs, discount rates and profit similar to what most practices experience.

The analysis of each plan will help the office staff to track, analyze and develop strategies that will enhance managed care in the practice.

How Payment Effective is the Managed Care Plan?

PLAN	# OF PATIENTS	CHARGES	ADJUSTMENTS	NET REVENUE	COST PER PATIENT	NET REVENUE PER PATIENT	PROFIT
A	100	$10,000	$2,500	$7,500	$75.00	75	0
B	700	$105,000	$31,500	$73,500	$75.00	105	$21,000
C	250	$50,000	$15,000	$35,000	$75.00	140	$16,250
D	250	$37,500	$15,000	$22,500	$100.00	90	($2,500)
E	1,000	$200,000	$80,000	$120,000	$90.00	120	$30,000
F	350	$78,750	$15,750	$63,000	$100.00	180	$28,000

PLAN	# OF PATIENTS	CHARGES	ADJUSTMENTS	NET REVENUE	COST PER PATIENT	NET REVENUE PER PATIENT	PROFIT
A	100	$10,000	$2,500	$7,500	$75.00	75	0

Plan A:

- The plan has a twenty-five percent (25%) discount rate.
- The cost, per patient, to provide $100.00 in medical care is $75.00.
- The practice does not earn a profit.

Strategies:

- Work with the physicians to find ways to reduce the cost per patient.
- Negotiate with the plan to reduce the discount rate.
- Terminate the contract.

PLAN	# OF PATIENTS	CHARGES	ADJUSTMENTS	NET REVENUE	COST PER PATIENT	NET REVENUE PER PATIENT	PROFIT
B	700	$105,000	$31,500	$73,500	$75.00	105	$21,000

Plan B:

- The plan has a thirty percent (30%) discount rate.
- The cost, per patient, to provide $150.00 in medical care is $75.00.
- The practice earns a profit on the plan.

Strategies:

- The net revenue per patient should be targeted for improvement.
- Work with the physician(s) to find ways to reduce the cost per patient.
- Negotiate with the plan to reduce the discount rate.

PLAN	# OF PATIENTS	CHARGES	ADJUSTMENTS	NET REVENUE	COST PER PATIENT	NET REVENUE PER PATIENT	PROFIT
C	250	$50,000	$15,000	$35,000	$75.00	140	$16,250

Plan C:

- The plan has a thirty percent (30%) discount rate.
- The cost, per patient, to provide $200.00 in medical care is $75.00.
- The practice earns a profit on the plan.

Strategies:

- The net revenue per patient is very strong.
- Work with the physician(s) to find ways to reduce the cost per patient.
- The practice should work with the plan to increase the number of patients.
- Negotiate with the plan to reduce the discount rate.

PLAN	# OF PATIENTS	CHARGES	ADJUSTMENTS	NET REVENUE	COST PER PATIENT	NET REVENUE PER PATIENT	PROFIT
D	250	$37,500	$15,000	$22,500	$100.00	90	($2,500)

Plan D:

- The plan has a forty percent (40%) discount rate.
- The cost, per patient, to provide $150.00 in medical care is $100.00.
- The practice loses money on the plan.

Strategies:

- Work with the physician(s) to find ways to reduce the cost per patient.
- Negotiate with the plan to reduce the discount rate.
- Terminate the contract.

PLAN	# OF PATIENTS	CHARGES	ADJUSTMENTS	NET REVENUE	COST PER PATIENT	NET REVENUE PER PATIENT	PROFIT
E	1,000	$200,000	$80,000	$120,000	$90.00	120	$30,000

Plan E:

- The plan has a forty percent (40%) discount rate.
- The cost, per patient, to provide $200.00 in medical care is $90.00.
- The practice earns a profit on the plan.

Strategies:

- The net revenue per patient should be targeted for improvement.
- Work with the physician(s) to find ways to reduce the cost per patient.
- Negotiate with the plan to reduce the discount rate.

PLAN	# OF PATIENTS	CHARGES	ADJUSTMENTS	NET REVENUE	COST PER PATIENT	NET REVENUE PER PATIENT	PROFIT
F	350	$78,750	$15,750	$63,000	$100.00	180	$28,000

Plan F:

- The plan has a twenty percent (20%) discount rate.
- The cost, per patient, to provide $225.00 in medical care is $100.00.
- The practice earns a profit on the plan.
- The net revenue per patient is very strong.

Strategies:

- Work with the physician to find ways to reduce the cost per patient.
- The practice should work with the plan to increase the number of patients.
- Negotiate with the plan to reduce the discount rate.

Evaluation of the managed care plan is a continuous process. The practice must constantly analyze, evaluate, and review the services, referrals, information, and reimbursement to determine if it fits within the goals and objectives of the practice.

Re-evaluate the Managed Care Plan

Step I. Information.

- What are the requirements to participate in the plan?
- How is the communication (verbal and written) with the plan?
- What is the time frame to obtain approval/certification?
- What is the growth trend for the plan (members, employers)?
- Is the Explanation of Medical Benefits (EOMB) user friendly — does it allow the practice to track payments, adjustments, and withholds?
- How are patient participants added? If capitated, do rates change with patient pool change?

Step II. Referrals.

- What are the managed care guidelines?
- Must the physician and/or staff call for authorization?
- Is there an updated listing of referring physicians?
- Who determines what services are considered medically necessary?
- Who is financially responsible for out-of-plan referrals?

Step III. Services.

- According to the managed care contract, what services will the physician be required to provide?
- What services are reimbursable?
- What services are not reimbursable?
- How do the reimbursement levels compare to other payers?
- What is the reimbursement trend (decreasing, increasing)?

Step IV. Reimbursement.

- What is the turnaround time for claims payment?
- How does the office know to collect co-pays and deductibles?
- What is the discount rate given by the managed care company? How does it compare with other payers?
- Is electronic filing an option?
- What is the appeal process?

CHAPTER 6

Cost-effective Health Care

Providing quality, cost-effective health care is the central issue. Though changes are in process, few physicians in training are exposed to managed care philosophies and the case management approach to patient care. In the academic setting, the focus is often on the care of the critically ill and patients with rare diagnoses. Residents are taught to be thorough and exhausting in their diagnostic journeys, and to rely on sophisticated technologies with limited consideration of the cost of these methods.

The gap between what is taught and what is expected of physicians today has become increasingly apparent as more physicians enter managed care organizations directly from residency programs. Many integrated delivery systems, MCOs and professional organizations are offering courses on managed care to meet the demands of the market.

This section will present some of the basic principles of cost-effective care for practice application.

Physician Education: The Key to Promoting Cost-effective Care

Although good medical care will never be inexpensive, there is much that can be done to lower costs without compromising quality. The adage that "quantity is not equal to quality" holds true in today's technologically advanced environment. Physicians are responsible for providing and ordering virtually all of the testing and prescriptions received by patients. Consequently, information regarding the cost of these services will be important to consider.

- *Learn the costs of the tests you order.*

    Hospitals, freestanding ambulatory centers, independent laboratories and diagnostic imaging centers can provide you with their charges for the services they offer. Catalog the most frequently ordered tests and obtain pricing information from these vendors. Have in your office lists to refer to when ordering tests. Know what potential alternatives are available to you that may be more focused and less expensive than a broad survey instrument. Be judicious; order only what needs to be done.

    Question your patients about tests they may have had recently that can be used rather than ordering new or duplicate tests. When your patients are tested, be certain that copies of the results are sent to your office, even when ordered by another practitioner. Maintain a complete file of current information.

- Keep accurate, detailed medical record documentation—both in your office and in the patient's acute care hospital record.

- Document why you are pursuing a particular clinical course, and your long-term follow-up plan. For quality care, it is essential to have appropriate chart documentation stating your thoughts about the case. It is more beneficial for you and your patient than excessive testing, which may yield only incremental information.

- Hospital based physicians should become familiar with reimbursement schedules. Testing rarely yields additional reimbursement for the hospital and/or the physician. Increasingly, predetermined fee scales and utilization reviews are integrated into the fee-for-service reimbursement system.

- Educate your patients on the type of testing you are ordering and why. Often, patients are more compliant and cooperative when they have a voice in their care and are informed about the risks and benefits of all procedures.

Practice Guidelines

Guidelines for a variety of clinical conditions are produced by many professional organizations, government agencies, and health care providers. It is important for physicians to be actively involved in the development of these guidelines. Guidelines are often the basis for future policy decisions and have an important impact on the practice. Be familiar with what group determines practice guidelines in the hospital and managed care organizations so you can be certain these efforts are led by physicians.

Studies examining the impact of guidelines on costs have shown that substantial reductions in use of resources has occurred with no demonstrable adverse effect on quality care. Therefore, be assured this method of care management will continue and become a stronger force in care delivery. The investment of your time and counsel in these processes is extremely important.

When reviewing managed care plans, ask for copies of their guidelines and question how those guidelines are formulated and what "rules for use" surround them. Will these be part of how you are "profiled" within the plan? Are their competing guidelines on the same issues from multiple plans?

Practice guidelines continue to proliferate. Physicians should insist the MCOs coordinate their guidelines development and implementation so the "rules" are not different based on individual payers. All patients should stand to benefit from the guidelines. Guidelines should not create competitive advantage for health care plans, but should create better methods of delivering care to all patients.

Information Sharing

Most, if not all, MCOs compare physicians with their peers in the area of resource utilization and practice patterns—a process called "profiling." Sharing this information to further the development of guidelines, critical pathways and recommended treatment protocols improves quality and lowers costs. Through information exchange and their response to it, physicians are participating in continuous quality improvement. It is important, however, that information exchanges are presented constructively and not used for "economic credentialing." Learn how data is presented and how individual physician profiles are shared (and with whom). Understand what information the MCO shares with other parties, for what purpose and in what form.

There are obvious benefits to the sharing of information as physicians and hospitals work together to improve the process of care. The coordination of this information is essential in that payers are increasingly requiring MCOs and hospitals to provide performance and cost data. The gathering of data is expensive, duplication is unnecessary, sharing and coordination will result in a system built on a foundation of appropriate resource utilization and continuous quality improvement.

Economic Analysis

There are many studies regarding the economics of health care delivery.

- *Cost identification studies* help determine the cost of a particular course of treatment. These are generally basic studies that consider a particular disease entity or DRG and track the treatment costs. They are generally only concerned with the dollars involved and often do not consider outcomes.

- *Cost effectiveness studies* are useful in comparing one type of medical intervention to another. They should be considered in isolation from other treatment options. The concepts of efficacy, effectiveness and efficiency must be addressed. In this type of study, efficacy refers to whether the product or intervention works under ideal circumstances. Effectiveness refers to whether that product or intervention works under "real world" conditions. Efficiency is whether the best outcome is obtained for the money spent. Often an "incremental analysis" is done simultaneously looking at additional costs and additional comments from alternative interventions.

- *Cost benefit analysis* is an attempt to report both costs and outcomes in economic terms. If the benefits outweigh the cost, the intervention in question is likely to be seen as a useful clinical strategy. Fallacy in this analysis (as in many analytical discussions in health care) is the difficulty of translating an outcome (such as the ability to live one year longer) into monetary value.

Though a variety of economic analyses can be used in considering the most cost-efficient manner in which to manage a particular case or disease entity, it is essential to understand the point of view of the study. There are generally four recognized points of view: (1) society's; (2) the patient's, (3) the payer's, and (4) the provider's. The point of view may have a dramatic impact on interpretation. For example, lowering the length of an inpatient hospital stay may substantially reduce the cost of care to the hospital (the provider). However, if the patient is unable to care for him or herself, the costs are merely shifted to the patient and his or her family.

Formal analysis aside, perhaps the best guidance available about efficient approaches to cost-effective health care delivery can be obtained by learning what your colleagues are doing and what the standard of care is in any given situation.

Medical Resource Management

Medical resource management studies focus on the efficiency and effectiveness of care delivery. There are generally three steps in this process.

- *Identification of priorities.* In determining what areas of study to concentrate on, high volume, high cost or high risk or high variance admissions or procedures may yield the most useful information.

- ***Data analysis methods.*** Data can be organized by hospital, department, diagnosis, ancillary service, or physician.

- ***Develop alternatives.*** Alternatives to consider might include the development of suggested clinical pathways for selected diagnoses; the implementation of specific policies or guidelines that monitor selected diagnostic tests, treatments, or procedures; or intensified concurrent utilization reviews that focus on the appropriateness and effectiveness of the treatment plan.

    There are computer programs currently being developed that allow electronic "scenario planning" for a variety of treatment protocols. While this type of analysis will never replace the role of the physician, it can create some stimulating thoughts for consideration.

    Computer generated order entry systems that include "real time" feedback education screens provide reminders of the costs and indications for certain tests and information regarding the appropriate utilization of antibiotics can promote and facilitate positive change.

Physician and provider input is continually elicited and conclusions are reinforced through ongoing education and monitoring. If the MCO you are considering or participating in does not have a significant physician involvement, find out why they do not include physicians. Carefully consider your choices regarding participation.

Outcomes Measurement

Measures to produce cost-efficient care include the formation of teams to provide a collaborative framework for improving the process of care. Data from many sources are collected and resource management steps applied. Surveys are used to evaluate patients' perception of the health care intervention. Practices are surveyed for outstanding processes and results. Data is organized and integrated into a format for delivery to physicians' office and/or hospital departments to improve the process, quality and cost effectiveness of care. Outcomes measurement processes are in their beginning stages. Physicians are in a key position to involve themselves in the design of these measurement projects.

Following outcomes measurement, we must be concerned with outcomes management. The questions are what to do with the data, how to influence wide scale process changes, etc.

In summary, cost-effective health care delivery can be approached from a variety of methods, education and use of data being primary to the process. It will be up to you, as a physician, to ultimately select the best approach for your individual patient, using the information available to you.

CHAPTER 7

Capitation Payment Systems

To fully look at capitation systems, understand their impact and develop your strategy, it is important to clearly understand what it is and how it works. This section provides that basic knowledge and stimulates your consideration of capitation issues in your own practice. It is not meant to be an exhaustive treatise on the issue, but serves more as a primer in this area.

In its basic form, capitation refers to an agreement to provide a certain range of services in exchange for a certain dollar amount. On the surface it seems fairly straightforward. The difficulty, however, comes in how well you are able to determine what are the services to be provided and in what amounts (i.e., patient utilization). This is the reason capitation systems are risk-bearing systems for the provider.

Though the payment per member per month (PMPM) is often adjusted according to age and gender, it is important to clearly understand the scope of service being required of you/your colleagues. This applies in both office and hospital settings. (Most capitation systems cover both office and hospital inpatient services.) You can obtain actuarial analysis of the potential risk. Consider this risk in light of your patient population (or the new population you will be taking care of under the contract), your practice style, and the actual costs you incur in rendering service.

The financial aspect of a capitation system is one that must be fully considered and one that will be affected by your ability to manage your patient population. This is often where physicians who are new to capitation systems have problems. Take the time to consider how you are going to respond to patient requests for technology and specialists that you may not feel are medically necessary at the time. What type of telephone triage system is operative in your office? Talk with your staff about their roles in responding to the needs of patients, either in person or over the telephone. How will the colleagues in your practice handle these same issues? It is the "soft" analysis that will have as much or more bearing on how successful you are in a capitated system than a percentage or two on the premium dollar.

When thinking about both the "soft" and concrete aspects of caring for a capitated population, consider the amount of staff needed to manage the data and billing requirements of the MCO, in addition to the care needs of your patients. Are there services you could provide in your office that you now have to refer to others? If so, what is the cost of the equipment and the training necessary to gear up to deliver this service?

Learn whether the MCO plans to "subcapitate" specialists and who makes up that panel of providers. Are some of the dollars for subcapitated specialists (most often ophthalmology, general surgery, cardiology and radiology) coming out of your monthly capitated amount? What risks are the subspecialists assuming and what risks are yours? If the patient has to be hospitalized and receive care by a subspecialist, what financial risks are you incurring for this event? What does the subspecialist plan for follow-up care to the patient and how is that paid for? What is your medical opinion of your colleagues on this panel and are you comfortable referring your patients to them?

Though capitation, in its earliest form, related only to primary care physicians, we are all aware it is also affecting the subspecialists. The table below illustrates the impact of capitation on specialists in a sub-capitated system.

COMMERCIAL	AVERAGE NON-MEDICARE REVENUES TODAY	TYPICAL COMMERCIAL PER MEMBER/PER MONTH	NUMBER OF CAPITATED LIVES NEEDED TO STAY "EVEN"
General Surgery	$329,736	$1.101	24,957
OB/GYN	$431,335	$2.305	15,594
Orthopedics	$487,564	$1.159	35,056
Radiology	$342,747	$1.910	14,954
Urology	$261,311	$0.497	43,815
MEDICARE	AVERAGE MEDICARE REVENUE TODAY	TYPICAL MEDICARE PER MEMBER/PER MONTH	NUMBER OF CAPITATED LIVES NEEDED TO STAY "EVEN"
General Surgery	$169,864	$4.624	3,061
OB/GYN	$32,965	$2.282	1,204
Orthopedics	$133,537	$5.447	2,043
Radiology	$160,553	$7.640	1,751
Urology	$206,989	$3.578	4,821

Source: The Health Care Advisory Board of Washington, D.C., based on information from the American Medical Association, Warren Surveys and Tillinghast Actuarial and Consulting Firm, 1994, The Advisory Board Company.

Another consideration relates to the care of the women patients in your population. Some may elect to see an obstetrician/gynecologist for pregnancy and an annual examination all though they are "your" primary care patient. Do you reside in one of the ten states who, by law, mandates access to OBs, physician assistants, or nurse practitioners specializing in care of women without a referral from the primary care provider? Again, who is on that panel? How does the payment work? What risks do you assume?

Capitation, as you are well aware, goes far beyond the definition of the term and quickly into your style and philosophy regarding patient care. Capitated care is not poor care; it is tightly managed care. In a capitated system, as a primary care provider, you are charged with that management.

Understanding this, please consider the information that follows in determining your costs and strategies relating to care provision. Again, you are encouraged to talk with your colleagues who have experience in the managed care arenas and learn from their experiences.

Having a working knowledge of the concept of capitation is a prerequisite for surviving and winning in a managed care environment. Following are the fundamental principles you will need to know and understand.

Basic capitation. Capitation is a prospective payment system that prepays a fixed dollar amount to contracting physicians, typically on a monthly basis. The amount is based on the MCO's determination of the cost of providing covered medical care for an MCO member for a month. Market factors also affect levels of capitated payment. *A physician accepting a capitated payment arrangement commits to providing the agreed upon primary care or specialty services for individual MCO member for a fixed dollar amount.* If no services are necessary for a particular member in a month, the physician still receives the capitated payment. However, if a member for whom the physician accepts a capitated payment requires an unusually high level of services in a month, there is no additional payment.

Capitated payment systems significantly change the nature and degree of the risk assumed by the physician. *In a capitated system, a physician is paid for the ability and commitment to provide medical services, not for the volume of medical services actually provided.* Some important points and ***advantages*** to remember are:

- Healthy patients (the low utilizers) are equally important as sick patients in a financial analysis of capitation.

- Capitation is paid to primary care physicians based on the number of MCO members who select or who are assigned to the physician for primary care for care management (care coordination or gatekeeping) services during the given month.

- Capitation is normally paid to other specialists based on the number of MCO members for whom the subspecialists are responsible.

- Capitation offers physicians a consistent, prepaid revenue stream. It encourages efforts to improve patient satisfaction and continuity of care so that patients will have a strong incentive to remain with the practice.

- Theoretically, capitated payment systems should reduce billing paperwork. However, most MCOs require a degree of information that may amount to almost as much encounter data as would appear on a fee-for-service bill.

The principal ***disadvantage*** of capitation is ***financial risk.*** Following are examples:

- The risk of the cost of medical care is placed on the provider. Sometimes these risks vary with circumstances over which the provider has little or no control; e.g., catastrophic illnesses or trauma, unfavorable patient mix, etc.

- While the transfer of risk may mean less direct intrusion by the MCO in clinical decision-making, it does require stricter operation and clinical controls by the physician. In particular, management information and cost accounting systems must be put in place to deal with these changes. The capital costs of these systems can be high. There is concern also, with the number of MCOs and their requirements, that they will not coordinate information needs and information management will become more burdensome.

Financial risks assumed under capitation can be limited or controlled by various mechanisms, such as stop-loss insurance.

Capitation can occur in many contexts. The following are common:

- An IPA or medical group may be paid on a capitated basis "on the front end," while individual physicians in the group or IPA can also be paid by capitation or may be paid on some type of discounted basis for service basis "on the back end." Depending on the make up of the group, capitation could cover only primary care services designed to be provided by the group, or primary care and other specialty services. This can occur even if the group does not have a full panel of specialists.

- An integrated delivery system might receive true global capitation by contracting to provide all medical care, including primary care, specialty care, inpatient and outpatient services, and ancillary services for a flat capitated amount.

- In a network or direct-contracting model HMO, an individual primary care physician might receive capitation only for primary care services, with all other services remaining the responsibility of the network or the MCO itself.

Ideally, MCOs use sound actuarial methods to determine capitated rates, using the same process as insurance companies to set their premiums. The methods are complicated and require the services of highly trained and skilled professionals. In reality, less precise methods or marketplace considerations often are used. At base, however, the process involves estimating utilization and cost of services covered by the capitated arrangement. This estimate may be based on actual historical data or on more abstract data, such as general industry-wide or population-wide statistics or demographic information.

In setting its premiums for members, the managed care organization adds its own profit and administrative costs to these estimates. The balance is allocated to the cost of medical services. For example, an MCO determines that on average each enrolled member will receive primary care services consisting of four office visits per year with one simple office lab urinalysis and with .5 electrocardiograms. The MCO budgets to pay $40 per office visit, $5 per urinalysis and $25 per electrocardiogram. This results in an annual expenditure of $160 for the office visits, $5 for the urinalysis, and $12.50 for the electrocardiogram, yielding a total budgeted expenditure of $177.50. To contract on a capitated basis, the MCO *would offer* to pay $14.79 per member, per month to a provider in exchange for a commitment to provide primary care services.

Utilization of medical services varies by age and by gender. Most managed care organizations vary capitation rates to distinguish between enrollees under age 65 (commercial members) and employees over age 65 (senior members). Some will also vary physician capitation by age and by sex among commercial enrollees. Capitation rates can vary by other factors, such as the characteristics of the group covered by a given capitation arrangement. Simply put, a group of office workers is likely to use fewer medical services than a group of factory workers. Experience can be adjusted based on actual experience of the group, or more frequently, on the standard industry classification codes.

When contracting for a capitation arrangement, having an exact definition of the scope of services included within the capitation payment is crucial.

- Avoid generically defined services such as "all services customarily provided in primary care," with few specific examples. This approach places the physician at a disadvantage in the event of dispute about what is and is not included in the flat fee capitation arrangement.

- Be specific, using phrases and codes from recognized sources such as the American Medical Association publication *Current Procedural Terminology, Fourth Edition* (CPT-4).

There are several specific risk factors that physicians should consider in capitation arrangements:

- **Panel size.** Larger patient panels reduce risk. The more MCO members assigned to a physician, the more the law of averages will protect the physician against catastrophic cases. The more patients — sick or well — choosing or assigned to a physician in a capitated arrangement, the more monthly revenue the managed care agreement will generate. The more monthly revenue a managed care arrangement generates, the less one or more patients with significant medical problems needing higher than anticipated care can affect profitability.

- **Adverse selection.** Adverse selection is when a panel of enrollees is heavily weighted by chronically ill patients as opposed to well patients or a more advantageous balance. Adverse selection is a particular problem for specialists and subspecialists entering capitated arrangements for primary care.

  - Adverse selection can be compounded for subspecialists when MCOs restrict or prohibit specialists or subspecialists from providing subspecialty care to their own patients, even if they are qualified to render that care, without going through a referral authorization process.

  - Physicians who seek to attract capitated enrollees from their existing practice may suffer adverse selection to the extent they are seeking patients only from a population already needing medical services. For the law of averages to work, the patient pool must include a representative number of individuals who need little or no medical care.

- **Over-marketing by the managed care organization.** Primary care physicians are vulnerable to MCOs that over-market their services or do not design insurance benefits appropriately. HMOs, in particular, stress preventive care. Individuals who market MCOs may assure patients that they can receive "all the medical care they want," in exchange for a flat premium. This can result in pressure from patients on primary care physicians to perform more services than are needed or were considered in the utilization assumptions on which capitation is based. Deductibles and copayments serve an important function in discouraging over utilization of office visits, particularly office visits for preventive care. In addition, physicians should review and monitor MCO marketing materials to ensure that they are not creating unreasonable expectations in the patient population.

- **Insolvency.** Insolvency as a managed care organization licensed as an HMO is a particular problem. All states regulate HMOs, and such regulations typically contain requirements called "hold harmless" provisions. In effect, those requirements bar a physician from seeking payment directly from any HMO enrollee, even upon nonpayment or insolvency by the HMO. Although they are required, as a condition of licensure, to have adequate reserves, some HMOs fail. Hold-harmless requirements reflect a balancing by state legislatures of the interests of the patient against the interests of physicians.

Risk pools. Risk pools vary greatly among capitated arrangements. There are shared risk pools for hospital and related institutional costs and a specialty (consultant) risk pool for specialist (consultant) costs. These two types of risk pools provide a way for physicians to receive an additional financial benefit from participating in a system that provides cost-effective care.

The operation of risk pools is illustrated best by working through an example. Where capitation is established for primary care services, but not for subspecialty or hospital services, the MCO will establish a separate fund or pool. The insurance organization, physicians, and other providers may participate in these pools. If a primary care physician receives capitation of $12 per member per month, $15 per member per month might be paid separately or allocated to the pool to pay for specialty (consultant) medical services, and $30 might be added to an "institutional" shared pool to pay for inpatient or institutional services and outpatient services. The primary care physician does not receive any of the money in the shared risk or the specialty (consultant) pool; it is held directly by the plan or IPA, sometimes in a separate trust account, and used to pay expenses appropriately charged to the pool. Non-primary care medical expenses paid out of the pool for members assigned to the primary care physician will be deducted from the pools. At the end of the year, a reconciliation is made. There may be some medical services for which the primary care physicians are not at risk through the referral or institutional services pool. For example, many MCOs negotiate a specific laboratory contract that requires all referrals to be made to that laboratory. Charges for laboratory services—either negotiated or actually determined—would be "backed out" of the pool. Only if a primary care physician orders a laboratory test from a different vendor will the charge be deducted from the pool. If, after the year-end reconciliation there is money left in a pool, some or all may be paid to participating physicians. If there is a deficit, participating providers *may* be required to pay—directly or through offsets of future fees—a portion of the deficit. These considerations should be clearly listed in the contract with the MCO, and the physician should review these clauses carefully.

In evaluating any risk pool participation, consider several factors:

- Risks can be both positive and negative. Participation in a risk pool can obligate a physician to pay if actual costs exceed the amount assigned to the risk pool. In most circumstances, this is modified contractually. Particularly for utilization of institutional services, it is often possible to negotiate a risk pool arrangement in which some participation in the upside of the risk pool will be available to the contracting physician without any obligation to participate in a downside.

- Risk pools can include physicians in one area or institution or physicians in several areas or institutions. *Generally, the more local a risk pool is, the more the practice patterns of a single contracting physician and those of similarly situated and similarly motivated physicians can hold down costs appropriately and ensure a financial return from the risk pool.* The more a risk pool is regionalized, or includes physicians in a variety of practice settings, the less any single physician or group of physicians is likely to have the motivation or means to encourage overall cost-effective medical practice.

- Risk pool accounting is usually performed by the managed care organization. It is important for contracting physicians to understand the mechanism for assigning costs to the risk pool. Having some right to audit the risk pool and returns made from it is also significant. Issues relating to expenses incurred but not reported are important in this context.

- In some managed care plans, a surplus in the specialist (consultant) pool or in the shared risk pool is used to defray excess expenses in the other pool. If specialist (consultant) referrals were more than the amount set forth in the specialist (consultant) risk pool, but institutional services were below the amount in the shared risk pool, funds available in the institutional services would be used to defray the excess in the specialist (consultant) pool. Many plans impose some limits on this inter-pool transfer, particularly by making only a percentage of the funds in the shared risk pool available to defray excess costs in the specialist (consultant) pool.

Withholds and bonus payments. Managed care organizations also commonly use withholds or bonus arrangements with risk pools. Withholds consist of a percentage withheld from fees otherwise due the physician. These withheld funds are typically used to pay excess expenses for services associated with that pool. Usually, after the expenses are paid, excess money is paid to participating physicians. However, there can be deductions and withholds that are not always paid back.

Address these issues related to distributions from these risk pools and unused withhold amounts:

- Determine which physicians are in a common risk pool. Aggregating physicians within one risk pool places one physician or group at risk for the practice patterns of another physician or group over whom there is little control.

- The manner for paying excess funds to physicians is also subject to considerable variation. In some arrangements, only physicians who have positive balances in the risk pools in which they participate receive any return. In other cases usually for primary care physicians individual physician risk pools are established, particularly for referral services. Funds may be distributed among physicians with a positive balance on a prorated basis or based on utilization and measurements of quality and member satisfaction.

- Incentive bonus plans offered to physicians are usually tied to patient satisfaction, quality of care as measured by the MCO, and cost-effectiveness. Typically, a composite of these ratings will be compared to the ratings of other physicians in the same risk pool. Cost-effectiveness may be measured in a variety of ways, but usually involves comparing the primary care physician to others in the risk pool, using actual costs per member per month. Many incentive plans are provided on a stratified or tiered basis. In such plans, physicians with the highest score will receive greater bonus awards than physicians with lower scores. For example, physicians in the top 75 percent of cost-effectiveness may be eligible for a bonus while physicians in the bottom percentage are ineligible. Those in the lowest percentages may even be candidates for termination from the managed care plan.

Accounting for expenses incurred but not reported (IBNR). The nature of referral and institutional services is such that there will be a lag between the time an obligation to pay for the service is incurred and the time the bill for the service is received and payment is made. This will always overlap the close of an annual accounting period for risk pools. These are commonly called incurred but not reported (IBNR) expenses. Monies otherwise available for distribution to physicians are withheld for payment of anticipated IBNR expenses. The methods of accounting for IBNR expenses are technical, but contracting physicians need, at a minimum, to assure themselves that proper historical data is used in projecting these expenses. Physicians should make sure that the IBNR estimate is included in the risk pool settlement accounting documents they receive and should track the ultimate, post-settlement payments for IBNR expenses to make sure the estimates were correct. In some circumstances, IBNR claims are not included in an annual settlement but are carried forward to a subsequent accounting period. Some MCOs provide periodic reports and even interim settlements or accountings of risk pool amounts.

Carve-outs. Carve-outs are a feature of many capitation arrangements and can take several forms. Certain services otherwise considered part of primary care for capitation purposes may in fact be provided through other arrangements. When this occurs, the services will be "carved out," both financially and definitely, from the capitated primary care arrangement. Carve-outs can also be used as a way to minimize the physician's financial risk for certain high-cost or high-risk medical services during the early period of a contract, to allow both the MCO and the contracting physician time to gain cost and utilization experience. In primary care, this type of carve-out is unlikely.

Capitation for subspecialists. Capitation for subspecialty services (e.g., cardiology, gastroenterology) poses the same set of basic issues as capitation for pure primary care services. Such capitation is normally calculated based on the number of patients in a population assigned to the subspecialist, as opposed to the number of patients who choose or are assigned to a primary care physician gatekeeper. Capitation for subspecialists is increasing in the marketplace. Direct capitation for subspecialty services may be encountered in MCOs organized along the IPA model, where a separate capitation budget is established by medical specialty, and subspecialists are held accountable for in-specialty results. Usually, in such a system individual subspecialists will still be reimbursed on a discounted fee-for-service basis with a fee withhold at risk for overall utilization within that specialty group. In addition, particularly for subspecialty services that are important but not used on a high volume basis, MCOs may pay capitated subspecialty reimbursement to a specific subgroup of providers. For example, a managed care organization might capitate a selected group of subspecialists in cardiology and require that all referrals from primary care physicians within a service area be made to those physicians. These arrangements are used, in particular, where a given market has an oversupply of certain subspecialists. One concern for physicians practicing a subspecialty is that this sort of virtually exclusive relationship may result in the practice becoming dominated by MCO referrals.

Percentage of premium reimbursement. Percentage of premium reimbursement is a managed care payment mechanism in which a fixed percentage of the health plan's premium dollars are prepaid to a medical group. Typically, this is on a monthly basis, based on the MCO's determination of the cost of providing covered medical care for a member for a period of time. At present, this type of reimbursement is not frequently encountered. Market factors also affect the levels of percentage-of-premium reimbursement that a managed care organization will pay. A physician group accepting a percentage of premium arrangement commits to providing an agreed bundle of services, to the extent necessary, to any individual member for whom the group receives a capitated payment. Often it is the responsibility of the medical group to find and pay for services that their patients need because the medical group has contracted to provide those services. This form of reimbursement has all the risk features of capitation with the added risk of errors in the rate-setting methodology employed by the MCO and its marketing efforts. The former could adversely affect physician fees if rates are set too low. The latter can adversely affect physician fees if the MCO is ineffective in its marketing. To the extent that MCOs undercut each other's premiums to capture market share, physicians accepting capitated payments on this basis will be helping to finance the effort.

Copayments and Deductibles. Contracting physicians are frequently required to collect copayments and deductibles from MCO members. Such fees play an important role in utilization management by discouraging MCO members from unnecessary utilization. Coinsurance, which may be required in an indemnity or fee-for-service managed care arrangement, necessitates a separate bill to the patient, normally after the MCO has determined an allowable fee-for-service payment amount.

CHAPTER 8

Capitation Strategies

Capitation Strategies — Multiple Issues, Multiple Approaches

Deciding on capitation strategies obviously includes not only the marketing of your practice, but determining your payment. This section provides information on a variety of ways to accomplish this task. One is primarily dependent upon actuarial data and the other, provided by J. Harper Gaston, M.D., President and CEO of Healthcare Partnership Consultants, Inc., Greenville, Georgia, is more prospective in nature as described below.

Both approaches should be considered as you look at the plan details, review the various approaches available to you and determine the most appropriate path. As you determine your payment, you should aggressively utilize this data in negotiating fees with the managed care organization as well as the length of the contract.

In his article, *Reflections on Ten Years of Capitation (Managed Care Medicine, September, 1995)*, Dr. Gaston relies on ten years of experience in developing capitation contracts for over 35 different physician specialties and subspecialties. He recommends using a reasonable cost-based analysis of both the business and support costs of the practice and simultaneously considering reasonable income by specialty and appropriate physician staffing ratios by specialty for a given population. Further, he cautions that *to be successful and competitive, it is imperative to obtain financially critical contracts (detailed in Table 2) before one assumes a major risk contract.*

It is also important to look at significant differences among the numbers of specialty physicians needed to care for Medicare, Medicaid and commercial members. Other considerations include office space, utilities, malpractice insurance and the like.

Dr. Gaston feels the aggressive actuarial approach offers only limited help in predicting the future changes and needs under managed care as it is more retrospective in nature. Further, his experience indicates that age and sex demographics are of limited value in nonprimary care specialties, though one must consider the separate capitation rates for Medicare, Medicaid and commercial enrollees in the specialty areas. If age and sex parameters are to be used, he recommends broad banding in 10–20 year brackets for non-Medicare and 5–10 year brackets for Medicare population. One guideline primary care physicians are offered is to negotiate for capitation rates at a level somewhat higher than the adult rate for children less than two years of age, and three to four times the adult rate for children two months of age and younger.

Table 1. Professional Commercial Capitation Rate Methodology.

Specialty	Physician/ Member Ratio	Physician Salary ($)	Physician Benefits ($)	Support Staff	Nonpayroll (35%) ($)	Other ($)	Total ($)	PMPM ($)†
Orthopedics	1 : 25,000	250,000	50,000	64,000	22,000	82,220	468,620	1.56
Ophthalmology	1 : 35,000	185,000	37,000	64,000	22,400	64,670	373,070	0.89
Internal Medicine	1 : 1,670*	132,000	26,400	70,000	24,500	36,750	289,650	14.45

*Three Primary Care Physicians per 5,000 members.
†PMPM = per member per month

Table 2. Capitation Rates Per Member Per Month for the Top Six* Physician Specialty Contracts for Each Category of Payment.

Specialty		Medicare ($)		Medicaid/AFDC ($)	
Primary Care	15.00	Primary Care	32.00	Primary Care	15.00
OB-GYN	2.90	Orthopedic	4.25	OB-GYN	5.75
Anesthesiology	2.50	Opthalmology	4.05	Anesthesiology	2.40
Psychiatry	1.75	Cardiology	3.50	Psychiatry	2.34
Orthopedic	1.40	Urology	3.50	Emergency Room	1.15
Emergency Room	1.18	General Surgery	3.10	Neonatology	1.00
Subtotal:	24.73 (65%)		50.40 (68%)		27.64 (85%)
Other †	14.12 (36%)		23.97 (32%)		4.70 (15%)
Total Professional	38.85		74.37		32.34

*These top six specialty contracts represent the majority of the total monies expended in each category of payment. (Commercial, $24.73 (64%); Medicare, $50.40 (68%); Medicaid, $27.64 (85%)).

†Of approximately 35 potential physician specialty contracts, only those six representing the greatest costs under each category of payment are given. "Other" represents the total capitation rates for the remaining 29 specialties.

There are at least 35 potential professional physician specialty contracts that could be obtained under capitation that makes expanding an organization's agreements seem to be an overwhelming task. As illustrated in Table 2, for commercial and Medicare members, this method suggests two-thirds of the monies can be controlled by implementing only six professional capitation contracts and for Medicaid, 85 percent of the monies can be controlled.

Dr. Gaston predicts a dominance of capitation payment mechanisms in the future. It is, therefore, essential that physicians begin now to accept capitation risk contracts while they may still have a fairly low mix of managed care patients in their population. This provides the experience necessary to thrive under these systems. "Physicians who understand capitation and can negotiate a fair capitation rate for themselves based on their own costs currently have a window of opportunity open to them."

Capitation Strategies — Another View

Turning capitation into a moneymaker requires thinking about patients, income, and expenses in new ways. While some practices are resisting change, others are making more money from prepaid care than they ever did from fee-for-service. There are two basic points to capitation strategy:

- To earn a profit, your costs must be less than the capitation payments.
- The risk you accept is commensurate with the patients *assigned* to you.

Third-party payers like capitation for three simple reasons. First, they pay a flat annual amount per covered life; second, it reduces their exposure; and third, their profit is established on the front end. With capitation, the insurers know what their cost is when they sell the contract. Their costs are the per member per month dollar amount that they allocate for doctors, hospital care, and administrative expenses. Their profit comes from the rate per member per month as sold to the employer less the cost.

The challenge to the provider is to know the administrative cost of providing the service to the patient. For the physician, there are many unknowns, so it is imperative to effectively use what financial information is available. Here is where to begin:

- Track by CPT code the number of times per year each service and procedure is performed, and what is billed for it. Analyze the corresponding RVS per CPT code to determine the prospective allowance.
- Armed with these statistics and your patient census, determine an average fee, utilization rate, and income per capita for your present practice.
- Since charges are often significantly higher than what is reimbursed, know your average reimbursement per CPT code, and by RVS.

Based on that knowledge, you can estimate a capitation rate for your practice. Beware if your fee schedule is too high (e.g., not linked to RVS or McGraw-Hill) or all capitation plans will seem unprofitable.

Be sure to collect the plan's copayments. If your office fails to take these collections seriously, this can cost you several ways. For one, the patient payments are a required part of your contract with the HMO; they serve as a disincentive from overutilizing your services, and that is important in capitation. Secondly, the copays are an important part of the practice's cash flow. Though each fee may be small, there is much revenue in the direct payment. Most HMOs ask patients to pay a $5 or $10 fee for each visit. If the plan is responsible for 1,000 patient visits a year, that is $5,000 to $10,000, and it may make the difference between profit and loss in your plan participation. Remember the following points:

- Collection of copays is required by the plan because it discourages over utilization. Capitation works best when patients get exactly the care they need, no more and no less.
- The dollars you collect from copays may be your profit margin on capitated contracts.

The plan's capitation figures are per thousand members, which includes those who will never come to your office. Your figures are based on how many services you performed — people you actually saw. The HMO may pay you less per thousand members than you would make per thousand patients, but some portion of those members will not cost you any office time. This makes the HMO the better bargain.

To bargain successfully on capitation rates, you must be prepared. Here are some helpful suggestions:

- With the help of an actuary, gather accurate utilization figures based on the total population involved. Beware of using the plan's own utilization figures as your only measure. The plan may be selective in how it interprets utilization, attempting to cast its rate in the best possible light.

- Using your computer system, start tracking some demographic data about your practice. Find out how many patients live in each surrounding ZIP code and their distribution by gender, age, diagnosis, and payer. (This requires a good billing system, plus a database or spreadsheet program that will allow you to import information from the billing software.)

- Set up your bookkeeping so you have the information you need to compare your current practice against capitation offers. Choose a medical-office computer-billing system that allows you to capture necessary data to track capitated arrangements. Systems that work best are similar to those used by TPAs (third party administrators). These systems are expensive and range from $50,000–$2 million. Some practices have pooled resources (often under an MSO) to obtain these services. Do not let the costs stop your analysis. A great deal can still be done with spreadsheet programs and the PC in your office.

- Look for the following features when looking for good managed-care capability in a computerized system.
    - It lets you enter all the discounted fee schedules by payer and assigns patient accounts to the appropriate plan, so the right fee schedules and copayments are automatically applied.
    - It records your outside referrals.
    - It lets you know whether you will meet the plan's goals for utilization.
    - It tracks referrals against corresponding utilization goals, so that you can appeal if the plan says you exceeded them.

- Ask about and understand the "withhold." (See Managed Care Descriptions.) To provide a financial incentive to keep costs to a minimum, most plans keep back part of the agreed-upon capitation payment. Before joining an HMO, ask if it has returned withholds and, if so, what percentage each year. Find out when withholds are distributed. Ask colleagues who are in the plan how promptly withholds usually have been distributed.

Besides tracking what kind of money you are making from HMOs, determine how much of your total income is coming from each payer. A basic rule of thumb is to not let any one plan represent more than 10 to 15 percent of your practice income. If you want more prepaid patients, join more plans. If a single insurer accounts for 25 to 33 percent of your income, it can assume too much control over your practice. As long as no single plan becomes overpowering, you can get out of any plan whose fee schedule conflicts with medical judgment or if the plan is not profitable to you.

Capitation forces a change in thinking about the way physicians are rewarded for providing more services. In capitation arrangements, profits depend on limiting utilization. In fee-for-service plans, a productivity-based income-distribution system is used. Therefore, a distribution plan must be set up that recognizes the value of meeting HMO utilization goals.

Here are some ways to do that.

- Assign each capitated patient a specific doctor, pay that doctor the capitation as it comes in, and charge all services for that patient against that doctor's income.
- A more complex scheme, use RVUs to determine the value of labor and services.

The key is to convert your internal bookkeeping to recognize the plan's utilization goals. Productivity is no longer the cash cow. That change is what makes capitation a challenge. The problem is that you may still think in terms of being paid more for seeing more patients and doing more for them. Capitation is the reverse of that. The transition makes things complicated.

CHAPTER 9

Determining Reimbursement

The next questions have to do with the managed care organization's payment structure. In short, what is the method of payment? Use of the following tools can help you gain valuable information for sound decision making.

Here's what you need to compare.

1. Enter the payment for Evaluation and Management procedure codes from the top three to five managed care plans.

2. Determine the relativity of the payer's payment on the codes. "Back out" the conversion factors for each code, using both the McGraw-Hill RVU and RBRVS. This will show you whether the payer lacks relativity between the procedures on its payment schedule.

- *Example* -

CPT Code	McGraw-Hill RVU	McGraw-Hill @ $5 Conv. Factor	Medicare RVU	Medicare @ $45 Conv. Factor	PPO#1 Payment	PPO#1 Medicare Conv. Factor	PPO#1 McGraw-Hill Conv. Factor
99211	6.5	$32.50	0.79	$35.55	$32.80	$41.50	$5.05
99212	9.5	$47.50	1.27	$57.15	$52.80	$41.50	$5.55
99213	14.0	$70.00	1.74	$78.30	$63.00	$36.20	$4.50
99204	20.0	$100.00	2.60	$117.00	$77.00	$29.60	$3.85
99215	26.0	$130.00	3.26	$146.70	$96.00	$29.45	$3.70

(Note: RVUs and Conversion factors are examples only.)

You can see by this example that PPO #1 is inconsistent in their payment. It's apparent that if the plan does use a Relative Value Unit Scale, it is not McGraw-Hill or RBRVS. You can use this information to investigate whether the payer used some other industry standard to arrive at the payment schedule. Note also whether the payer's conversion factors fit in with the range of conversion factors for that region.

As a final comparison step, look at the Explanation of Benefits (EOBs) from each managed care plan being used in the analysis. What is the historical plan payment? Does the plan pay at the contracted rate? You can pull much information from EOBs.

Determine the Weighted Average of the Plan

In addition to calculating conversion factors, and comparing fees against Medicare and contracted plans, determining the weighted average reimbursement for managed care plans can be useful when negotiating contracts. Weighted average means the percent of the physician's total charges for which he is reimbursed by the plans he participates in. Each plan's discount schedule may be different; therefore, a total of the plans provides a weighted average return; e.g., 83 percent of regular charges.

Look at the contracted plans one at a time. Using a weighted average calculation, target a specific goal for the percentage of reimbursement from payers. Here is how:

1. Complete Schedule B — (using the sample on the following page) with the following information for the most frequently billed Evaluation and Management and procedure codes.

    – Practice fee

    – Frequency the procedure is performed (annually)

    – Plan payment

2. Multiply both physician charges and payer reimbursements by the frequency these procedures are performed.

3. Calculate the total gross charges and total gross payments for all CPT codes.

4. Divide the total gross payments into the total gross charges to determine the weighted percentage of reimbursement for this plan.

Many practices have a target of 80 percent reimbursement on their fees. This is a good target figure, but often difficult to achieve in today's market. The setting of the fee schedule is critical as that is on what the 80 percent is based. One can afford to take less of a percentage of a higher fee schedule.

Determine the Weighted Average of the Plan

- *Example* -

CPT Code	Frequency	Your Charge	Gross Charges	Plan Payment	Gross Payments
99211	80	$45	$3,600	$36	$2,880
99212	47	$63	$2,961	$55	$2,585
99213	56	$65	$3,640	$52	$2,912
99214	20	$64	$1,280	$47	$940
99203	32	$81	$2,592	$66	$2,2112
99204	40	$128	$5,120	$111	$4,440
TOTAL			**$19,193**		**$15,869**
Weighted Average Reimbursement					**83%**
Discount					**17%**

Calculations:

- Total Payments / Total Charges = Weighted Average
- 100 - Weighted Average = Discount

(See Exhibit 9-2 for form, page 107)

CHAPTER 10

Marketing to the Managed Care Marketplace

Positioning in the Marketplace

Physicians who wish to position their medical practice in the marketplace must (1) understand how medical practices are evaluated by managed care organizations for initial contract and subsequent contract renewal; (2) assess the individual desires, market position, and strategy of each medical practice; and (3) take steps to demonstrate the desirability of the practice. MCOs judge medical quality in several ways:

- Focus on physician's credentials and background.

- Interviews by the MCO medical director, often in the physician's office or other practice setting.

- Requirements for physician licensure, hospital affiliation, and certification by the appropriate specialty boards.

- For those who are not board-certified, demonstration of individual training and experience to furnish equivalent evidence of qualification.

- Chart review in physicians' offices, using predetermined standards to document the appropriateness (by MCOs standards) of care. (See *How to Handle an Audit by an MCO*, page 84.)

- Site visits focusing on
  - cleanliness and accessibility
  - performance of office-based lab procedures
  - scheduling to determine the number of patients seen per day
  - lapse time between patient request and the appointment
  - the time between patient arrival and the physician encounter
  - provision of preventive care.

- Provider profiling (primary care) comparing performance based on specific norms. Often called "benchmarking," this process focuses on performance in terms of
  - total cost per case, average length of stay, readmission or complication rates for inpatient services
  - average cost per patient encounter, per diagnosis, average number of visits per member, per year
  - average utilization of ancillary services (including diagnostic tests, laboratory tests and imaging tests) together with average cost per encounter

- Review of physician practice patterns consisting of process reviews and focused reviews.
  - Process reviews include retrospective examination of specific cases, chosen randomly or because they involve specific procedures or a specific diagnosis, usually conducted by MCO employees.
  - Focused reviews entailing an in-depth evaluation of cases involving poor outcomes, unusual practice patterns or extraordinary results, conducted by the peer review process.

Practice Evaluation and Assessment

Positioning for managed care contracting involves a practice assessment. Similar to developing a managed care strategy, assessments should consider:

- Summary and review of patient geographics and demographics that reveal where the practice's patients live and work and what types of occupations, income levels, age ranges.

- Evaluation of what type of patients a medical practice is seeking and what geographical areas work well with the existing hospital, specialist, and ancillary service provider affiliations.

- Determination of the compatibility of a managed care contract with existing referral sources.

- Review of the existing marketplace for MCOs and competitive medical practices.

- Career plans and goals assessments in relation to physician's market stage and career stage.

- Assessment of tangible and intangible assets of the practice. Such assets include facilities and staff; administrative systems for cost accounting, billing and reimbursement; and existing or needed medical or computer equipment.

- Self-assessment of the physician's own ability to deal with the managed care environment.

Marketing to Payers and Employers

There are two levels of managed care marketing. First, individual physicians must market to existing networks or new networks in the formative stages to become a member of the organization. Second, physician network organizations must market themselves to potential payers and employers. At either level, accumulate and maintain as much available data as possible for use in marketing and contract negotiations. The following profile should be developed for use in negotiating contracts.

The Initial Physician Network Profile Package: Sample Contents

- A complete listing of the network's members, their specialties, and their geographic locations
- Each physician's hospital affiliations
- A map showing practice locations and delineating primary care and specialty practices, hours of operation, urgent care capabilities, etc.
- A description of the credentialing criteria

- A description of the organizational structure, management, and operational plan
- A description of the types of contracts wanted and the numbers, demographics, and geographic coverage of the populations it wishes to serve
- Commentary about willingness and capability to enter capitation and discounted fee-for-service contracts

This seems like a lot of data to gather, and it is. However, the keys to obtaining contracts you want and the patient mix that works best for your particular practice are to know where you are going and to work hard to get there. Informational packets such as the one described above will be invaluable to your practice. You can use this information as you recruit new physicians, introduce yourself to a new employer, introduce a new partner to the community, etc. To gather the information and take the time to present it in a friendly, solid manner will inure to your benefit many times over.

Here are what purchasers look for from health care provider networks:

- Multispecialty networks with a good balance between primary care and specialty physicians
- "Niche" single-specialty networks
- Networks that cover a wide geographic area and provide comprehensive services
- Networks that collaborate with efficient institutions
- Willingness to capitate
- Advanced capabilities in procedures, research, and treatment
- Ambulatory and preventive care activities and programs
- Commitment to value, quality, information systems, and self-regulation

Marketing in Managed Care

The fundamental marketing principle in the managed care era is: **make your practice attractive to managed care plans.**

Basically, this is accomplished by **providing high quality, low cost patient care** and achieving and maintaining **patient satisfaction.**

Although it may sound simple, if you are responsible for the health of people in large capitated pools, and an excessive number of patients have extended illnesses, you could suffer financially. So, how can you make a profit treating more patients at lower reimbursement without sacrificing quality of care?

Concentrate on Patient Satisfaction

- **Treat everyone the same.** It makes no sense to discriminate against your managed care patients. A two-tiered system of care within a physician's office is too cumbersome to maintain. Even if it achieved the desired results, the following problems could occur:
  - ethical dilemmas
  - the risk of being targeted for discrimination and/or malpractice
  - economic risk (e.g., loss of managed care contract(s))

- **Stress quality service.** That means seeing patients when they need to be seen. Managed care plans focus not only on cost, but on quality and patient satisfaction. Most plans conduct follow-up phone surveys with patients to determine their level of contentment with the services of the physicians and staff and to ascertain whether they have any suggestions or complaints they would care to make. Disgruntled patients might pressure employers to choose another plan.

- **Patient satisfaction translates to dollars.** In some plans, the bonus check at the end of the year is based on how well patients like your style of practice.

Know your contract down to the last clause. Know exactly what services are covered before entering the exam room. Otherwise, you could wind up providing services that will never be paid for or promising services that cannot be provided (through the plan). It is not a question of treating patients differently but knowing the boundaries dictated by the plan.

- Create a master form for each plan that lists its guidelines, copay, deductible, and other information.

- Have available, every time you see him, the information about your contractual obligation to this patient. Place a copy of the plan summary in each patient's chart if that is helpful. Be cautious, however, about labeling the outside of the chart with plan information. Though it may be a quick reference, it can make the patient wonder if he is receiving a different level of care based on the managed care plan.

- Before providing noncovered services, secure the written consent of the patient indicating the patient's understanding (1) of the service to be provided, (2) that the MCO will not pay for or be liable for the noncovered service, and (3) that the patient is liable for the payment of the noncovered service.

Adjust your appointment schedule to protect the practice. While it is not appropriate to limit the care you give a managed care patient, it may be appropriate to use scheduling strategies to maximize the number of patients (i.e., covered lives) you contract with from each plan. The rule of thumb in business is never allowing one income source to exceed 25 per cent of the total revenues for the practice. Control your mix of patients to avoid becoming vulnerable in the event of a contract termination. Most insurers can cancel their contract on 90 days' notice. Once you sign on, there may not be an option of turning away new patients. If you do that, the plan could drop you.

Reach out with midlevel providers. Consider using nurses, nurse practitioners, and physician assistants to free up your time. Not all patients need to be seen by the doctor and can be well cared for by midlevel providers. These providers often build a practice quickly and have strong patient loyalty.

- **Delegate.** Delegation is often difficult, but important. Make full use of midlevel practitioners. Discuss with them your expectations and learn about theirs. Determine their strengths and weaknesses, likes and dislikes and delegate appropriate patient services. They can provide a high quality service and generate appreciable revenue to the practice. Good midlevel practitioners who are under utilized and under challenged will not only be expensive, but will be difficult to retain.
- **Educate** patients and other staff about the services mid-level practitioners can provide. Market their talents within your practice. Set definite hours for them to work and clearly outline your expectations. Be available for questions and provide the required supervision. They can be a valuable part of the team if their roles are understood and appreciated.

Use the telephone effectively. Establishing a system of priorities for handling telephone calls is an essential element in managed care.

- Screen calls to identify those that can be directed to others such as calls put through immediately to the physician (emergencies, physicians and specific callers); returned calls (prescriptions, refills and test results); and calls handled by staff (nurses, administrators and billing).
- Patients often pressure staff members to answer questions and give advice. These calls should be handled by a reliable medically licensed staff member who is trained to distinguish between patients who need to come in for an appointment, those who can be seen by a midlevel provider, and those who need to be called back by the physician. When in doubt, nurses or assistants should consult the physician.
- Communication is what we say, how we say it and how well we listen. When office personnel are speaking with a patient by telephone, the patient can only relate to what they hear. Therefore, when patients need to be discouraged from making inappropriate office visits, diplomacy is important. Your designated staff member must be upbeat, friendly and helpful as they respond. One response might be to thank the patient for calling and to let them know that you can probably save them from a trip into the office.
- Document patient calls and clinical matters in the patient's chart. Include the date, time, substance of the conversation and the person taking the call. Note the nature of the complaint, and any medications being taken. Record what response or information was given, and place the completed message sheet in the patient's chart.
- Some patients will insist on seeing the doctor. When a patient insists on coming in, whoever takes the call should schedule the appointment and note the conversation in the patient's chart. Respond with flexibility if the patient wants to be scheduled soon. Otherwise, the patient may complain to the plan, or he may find someone else who will see him.
- Return all calls promptly. Encourage patients to call the office any time if their symptoms worsen. Provide the name of the designated staff member who handles calls and encourage them to contact this person first.
- Designate a time each day for returning calls. It is important to return all calls on the same day the patient called in.
- With a properly trained staff, good telephone medicine and patient education can be done when patients call in and describe their symptoms.
- Establish an after hours answering system, either by using an answering machine or answering service. If a machine is used, make sure your message provides a number where you can be reached in an emergency. For nonemergency calls, say that a doctor or nurse will

return the call as soon as possible. Avoid using messages that only give your office hours or directs the caller to dial 911. Neither should a patient be directed to the emergency room in an emergency.

If subscribing to an answering service, call periodically to see how patients are treated. Your answering service reflects the commitment to care just as much as the rest of the staff. Tell the answering service what the office requires to promote professional courtesy. If calls are not handled to your standards, find one that meets your expectations.

- State in your employee handbook that unauthorized personnel who gives advice or answers questions will be subject to immediate firing. Your reputation, your patient's safety, and your exposure to malpractice liability rely on the accuracy of the information your patients receive. In addition, if your managed care plan discovers that an unlicensed employee is giving medical advice, you are likely to be dropped from the panel.

Develop Written Guidelines for Prioritizing Calls.

Provide details about what type of advice staff members can give over the telephone. Such guidelines also establish how calls are handled. A telephone manual provides a degree of malpractice protection by providing evidence that employees are following your approved guidelines. Managed care plans view written guidelines favorably because of their interests in quality and patient satisfaction.

The following suggestions will help your staff confidently and appropriately handle calls.

- If you practice with other physicians, meet with them to discuss how to handle commonly encountered conditions and symptoms. Include your nurses in these discussions. Be united in your approach. Test the process for loopholes or vagueness.

- Include a section on telephone etiquette. Cover suggestions such as answering calls quickly, smiling when speaking, and placing calls on hold courteously. Emergency calls should never be put on hold.

- Set up a section on each condition or system that is frequently treated in your practice (e.g., ear, head, heart, nose, etc.). Include a short list of questions under each heading to obtain information about the patient's symptoms. Follow with your specific scheduling guidelines.

- The manual will be easier to use if subjects are alphabetized and pages are numbered. Use a three-ring binder for durability and ease of updating.

- Place a copy of the manual near each phone in the office.

- Instructions for handling medical emergencies must be posted prominently near each telephone. Include the telephone number of the local poison control center on this instruction sheet.

    - Route calls about chest pain, heavy bleeding, fainting, seizure, and poisoning to the physician immediately.

    - Direct the patient to the nearest emergency room if no doctor is available. Call an ambulance if the patient is unable to get there on his own. Arrange for a doctor to meet him at the hospital.

    - Obtain the caller's phone number in the event you are disconnected.

    - Test your procedures by using "mystery callers." Doctors or nurses can be used to simulate emergencies. By successfully completing these drills, your staff will develop a level of confidence.

Implementing these telephone protocols will help demonstrate to managed care plans the quality of service your practice provides. Monitoring patient outcomes also provides documentation on the quality of your services. Consider computerizing your clinical records to maintain outcomes so you can analyze the data.

Document and demonstrate patient satisfaction. As a provider of high quality, low cost patient care, it is important that you can demonstrate it. Distribute questionnaires to both your patients and their referring physicians to evaluate your staff and yourself. A biannual mailing to either the entire practice or a random sample is recommended. Or have phone surveys conducted to obtain feedback.

The Patient Satisfaction Survey (See Exhibit 10-1, page 109) covers the full spectrum of providers and services typically found in a physician's office or clinic. The survey should be given to the patient, by the physician, at the conclusion of the visit or mailed separately from any other information (e.g., monthly statement).

Results must be communicated, good and bad, with physicians and staff in a timely manner. Patients who are dissatisfied should be contacted and thanked for their suggestions/comments. A note in the chart of the problem may be useful to refer to on their next visit to assure them you have made note of their concerns.

Who is Marketing What to Whom?

We have discussed ways in which you can market yourself and your practice to the managed care marketplace. In turn, the MCO will be marketing its services and its network of providers to employers and other payers. To secure business in a highly competitive market, the MCO will be using traditional marketing skills along with "measurable data" which includes the performance of physicians in the network. Often called a "grading system" or "report card," this tool is quickly moving into third generation standards for measuring and reporting performance. You will be reviewed, "graded" and compared to your peers by the MCO as a part of their cost and quality assurance strategy. This also gives them an extra boost in promoting their managed care network to potential buyers.

It will be important to physicians to understand the grading system and to be active in assisting with its design and judging its effectiveness. The savvy physician will not simply point to the problems in the grading system, but will assume an active role in design and implementation.

There are two organizations you should become familiar with. One is the Health Plan Employer Data and Information Set (HEDIS) and the National Committee for Quality Assurance (NCQA). HEDIS is being developed through the NCQA. The NCQA is the leading accrediting body for managed care organizations.

The HEDIS information basically is acquired from hospital and physician data (through insurance claims) or through focused medical records audits. It consists of 28 technical measures and responses to eight questions on an enrollee satisfaction survey conducted independently. HEDIS considers such issues as immunization rates, preventive services, quality, access and patient satisfaction. These measures are considered to be in their infancy, and employers are not using them widely at this point due to concern about the accuracy of the data. However, it is coming. NCQA spent over $2,000,000 to fund a Report Card Pilot project in early 1994. This pilot utilizied voluntary MCOs along with a multidisciplinary group representing employer, consumer, health policy and labor representatives. The technical report suggests that plans, in the main, are performing well on most measures.

The real issue facing physicians, MCOs, and payers is in considering how the data is obtained, measured, reported and used. The data is not complete, and the premise upon which to base findings is hotly debated. The idea of a report card of some form, however, is inevitable. What demographic and socioeconomic factors skew data, e.g., the high propensity for asthma in inner city children; what impact does technology have on the outcomes measure; what utilization is optimal; how do gender and age differences figure in and complicate the issues; who decides on the "risk adjustment" and on what basis? These and thousands of other questions face those gathering, interpreting and being assessed.

As a physician in a managed care network, you should talk openly and candidly with the medical director of the plan regarding these issues. What is the data? How is it being used? What is the comparison group? How can you influence the data? When will you see it? What determinations are being made on it? How are employers influencing the choices made by their employees?

The answers to these questions and an active involvement will have multiple payoffs in the end. As you consider your information systems, consider the data you will be expected to submit in the next three to five years and in what format. In looking at coding issues within your office, it is essential, even more than ever before, to consider the accuracy of the coding decisions being made.

In short, while you are managing the care of your patients, be certain you are also allowing full consideration to managing your risk, your reputation and your ability to contract with managed care organization now and in the future. The key is active participation; the hazard lies in passive acceptance.

Tips to Market Your Practice and Increase Patient Satisfaction

Controlling utilization and increasing patient satisfaction while providing a high level of service is the key element to surviving and thriving in a managed care arena. The tips below should be helpful as you consider your individual approach to this challenge, keeping in mind that increasing your market share should yield lower costs overall. Most of these strategies are being practiced in a managed care environment in the United States. Depending upon where you reside, you may be providing these services or competing against them.

- Keep an accurate, up-to-date quality file in your office so it is readily accessible to you, your colleagues and in case of a visit from MCO. In this file, keep track of credentials, Certified Medical Education plans, certifications, staff meetings where quality is discussed, commendations, complimentary letters from patients and referral sources, office memos concerning quality, data from the hospital and other sources;

- Keep a file current with your Curriculum Vitae (reviewed and updated at least annually), copies of CME programs completed, CME plans for the future, notes of any committees you have or are currently serving on and your office or role, any work completed or in progress toward the AMA Physician Recognition Award;

- Audit your own charts in your office by having one of your staff members routinely (monthly) screen an agreed upon number of charts against criteria set by you and your colleagues. Be sure this information is discussed at your monthly staff meetings and make note of it;

- File your patient satisfaction surveys and results along with any action plans that have been formulated to address problems;

- Keep easily accessible records of your most common diagnoses, the hospitalization rates of your patients (and the reasons), your charges and reimbursement. By having someone in your office set up a table for this information and routinely compile it, you will be ahead of the game;

- Access any outcome studies available that compare you with your regional colleagues;

- Faithfully log information about your workers' compensation patients (their diagnoses, treatment plans, amount of time off work, etc.);

- Do not overlook patient needs for convenient locations, late or early office hours, weekend services, waiting time, follow-up, staff response, etc.

Studies have shown that patients who have or believe they have poor access to medical care will require more frequent and longer hospitalizations than those who avail themselves to routine and preventative care. Make your office a place that assures access and is committed to a high level of patient satisfaction.

There are practices that are currently —

- Making house calls;

- Routinely calling patients back to see how they are feeling and answer any questions;

- Keeping a "tickler" file for reminding patients by mail of the need for preventive services such as pap smears, mammography, etc.;

- Training triage nurses to function against a set of preapproved criteria in managing patients by telephone when appropriate;

- Offering clinics, either alone or with hospitals or other practices, in the areas of smoking cessation, diet, exercise, etc.;

- Providing health information services to local schools and churches;

- Utilizing physicians and other staff in an active speaking bureau to community organizations on a proactive, routine basis;

- Publishing newsletters on health care topics while profiling individual providers and announcing newly recruited physicians or newly begun services;

- Serving in a variety of public service and volunteer roles in their communities.

As the market gets even tighter and patient expectations grow, the need to be more proactive and deliberate will be essential to practice growth.

(See *Patient Satisfaction Survey*, page 109.)

How to Use a Patient Satisfaction Survey

- If you want patients to complete a satisfaction survey, be proactive in your request. Do not simply leave it at the desk. The person who registers patients or schedules follow-up appointments should give a copy to the patient and ask them to complete it before leaving or send it in soon. Include a stamped, business-reply envelope to maximize the number of surveys returned. Consider amending the format to at least collect the zip code on patients who do not wish to reveal their name and home address. This will be useful in your geographic analysis.

- Distribute a significant number of surveys so a statistical analysis has some meaning.

- Determine if you will survey quarterly, bimonthly, or semiannually. Then select certain weeks or a full month in that time when all patients will be asked to complete surveys. This should give you a good cross section of your patient base.

- Have one person in charge of data gathering, analysis and reporting of responses. This is often a role for the office manager.

- Be certain results are discussed in physician and full staff meetings within 60 days of the completion of the survey distribution. You will find it easier to recall and make changes on current data. Elicit change ideas from your staff.

- Number or otherwise code individuals who may be negatively referred to by name so the message is heard and the individual is protected. Share this information with that person or the lead physician so education can take place.

- Keep copies of the raw data and analysis for use in benchmarking progress and to better serve your patients in the future. Format the collected information in a way that it can be used for documenting results to your managed care plans.

- If your managed care organization requires a patient survey, try to combine your needs and theirs to one form so the data is useful to both.

- Be certain to follow up with unhappy patients by a phone call or in writing from the office manager or the physician. Dealing with dissatisfied patients forthrightly pays huge dividends in both the long and short run.

- Survey routinely to get the most from your efforts. Do not wait until there are problems or data deadlines. Develop and adhere to an annual survey schedule that meets your needs and that of your MCOs.

How to Handle an Audit by a Managed Care Organization

- From the outset, understand your contractual arrangement with the MCO and what your obligations are.

- Keep clear and accurate charts reflecting care given and your thoughts on the case over time.

- Be certain office charts are up-to-date and referral reports have been filed in a timely fashion.

- Note any phone calls between the physician and patient and/or the physician and MCO in the chart. When speaking to someone with the MCO, be sure to note their name and telephone number.

- Ascertain why the MCO is auditing your practice and if they are auditing other practices as well. Find out what they are looking for specifically so you can simplify the audit process. Explain any issues that result from the audit. Is the audit routine? Is there a problem? Has a patient complained?

- Talk with colleagues who may have undergone a similar audit and learn from their experiences.

- Find common ground. How can this audit improve patient care and/or your MCO relationship?

- Determine what the MCO will do with the information it gathers and if it has or will be filing reports with other agencies. If this is the case, what agencies and for what purposes?

- Keep a record of what information is requested, who made the request and when the information was provided. Keep all originals and send only copies. Check with the hospital (if the audit involves a hospitalized patient) to see what records have been requested from them and what they have sent to whom.

- Do not panic. Gather as much data about the audit and the reasons for it as you can. Be forthcoming with information. As possible, work with the MCO and not against it.

CHAPTER 11

A Word About Medicare and Medicaid

Like other areas of practice reimbursement, HMOs are having an increasing impact on Medicare and Medicaid populations. As of this writing, Congress is in the process of revamping the entire Medicare program as part of the budget reduction efforts. The final plan promises to be the result of protracted discussions over time, but will, in all likelihood encourage more seniors into managed care plans. Thus, the number of HMOs offering Medicare and Medicaid risk-contracting plans has grown rapidly and that growth is expected to accelerate.

Risk-contracting plans are the most common of the three managed care variations approved by the Health Care Financing Administration (HCFA) for seniors. Medicare risk-contracting is an arrangement between an HMO and Medicare in which the HMO receives a fixed monthly payment for the "covered lives" (e.g., Medicare Beneficiaries) enrolled. The HMO is at risk to provide all the medically necessary services for those "covered lives." The other plans are called "cost" and "health care prepayment plan" contracts.

Risk contracting plans require more comprehensive care for Medicare HMO patients. The "risk" factor is that: reimbursement in an HMO product is tied directly to your ability to provide cost-effective care.

Medicare Contracts

Although similar, there are subtle differences in Medicare HMO contracts and commercial contracts. Primary care physicians in a Medicare HMO typically are capitated and paid on a per member per month basis at a rate generally three to four times higher than on the commercial side. But the money is used quickly because seniors tend to have more medical problems and more frequent office visits.

There is also a geographic component to Medicare HMO reimbursement that could mean more or fewer capitation dollars. Using a formula known as adjusted average per capita costs (AAPCC), HCFA projects, on a county-by-county basis, what an average Medicare patient's care will cost. HCFA then subtracts five percent to come up with its payment to HMOs. The HMOs, in turn, base their capitation rates for physicians on what they get from the government. The assumption is that net income is leveled. This may benefit physicians who practice in a location with high Medicare fee-for-service costs, but it may penalize physicians in low-AAPCC counties (usually rural areas) whose Medicare HMO payments are far less generous.

Administratively, Medicare HMOs rely on preauthorization and referral rules. Seniors often need help understanding and following HMO rules, especially those who are accustomed to having a fee-for-service plan. Therefore, the practice can anticipate providing some new-member orientation to help Medicare patients understand what to expect in an HMO and to avoid future misunderstandings.

In Medicare HMOs, seniors can retire from one plan and enroll in another with only one to two months' notice. To change plans requires filling out a single form. This could benefit a physician who changes from one Medicare HMO to another. If the senior patient wants to stay with the physician, Medicare makes it easy for them to switch to the new plan.

The benefits covered by a Medicare HMO can be quite comprehensive and greatly exceed Medicare Part B benefits. Plans may offer seniors a wide array of services, especially in competitive markets, including some or all of the following:

- prescription drugs
- psychotherapy
- vision care
- hearing aids
- dental coverage

In Capitation, prevention pays

Although the payment mechanism is different, the care given to patients should not differ from Medicare Part B patients. However, caring for seniors in managed care is different from fee-for-service. Both prevention and aggressive case management are stressed, requiring a greater level of oversight and coordination by the primary-care physician. Patient-management skills are especially important in Medicare, because seniors use a wider array of services from multiple providers. Usually, care is delivered at a higher level of coordination, which benefits the patient. Though the populations are different, there are many similarities between managing Medicare and Medicaid populations. As appropriate, consider these measures for patients in both programs.

Managing care is vastly different from taking care of patients episodically. Here are some steps that may help in managing care:

- Ask each new patient to bring in all prescription medications. Eliminate unnecessary or potentially dangerous drugs and combinations that seniors may have picked up changing from doctor to doctor under fee-for-service.

- Send a midlevel provider, nurse, or social worker to a new patient's home to assess support systems and identify potential health hazards; occasionally, a doctor will also visit. Although this level of case management costs valuable time and money, it pays off eventually.

- Look for preventive measures that may require an up-front expense, yet eventually save money and time by preventing an injury to the patient. An example would be to buy a bathtub bar for a patient to prevent a fall resulting in a fracture. Reduce cost by working in the prevention stage rather than during the intervention stage.

Case management helps minimize the risk

Total case management is a highly developed skill. Keeping tabs on benefits from multiple providers is challenging. Establishing preventive routines, such as immunizations, is a part of the effort to become a good patient manager.

Risk contracts can be financially losing propositions. Such scenarios occur if you have a disproportionate share of high-utilizing seniors with multiple system diseases. Other losses can occur with at-risk populations in the child bearing ages (Medicaid) with multiple system diseases or lack of financial resources to secure adequate basic living requirements (i.e., food, housing, preventive care, transportation). Capitation rates are generally risk-adjusted by age and sex to counterbalance the cost increased by sicker patients. Still, to protect your practice, stop-loss insurance is recommended. This limits your liability for elderly patients who develop costly, catastrophic illness. This insurance is built into some HMO contracts.

You are at less financial risk if you are capitated only for the care you provide, because the HMO is not holding you accountable for high-priced specialty or inpatient care. But even primary care groups taking limited risk can lose money if seniors monopolize their time. Use your staff appropriately to do the following to minimize your time spent unnecessarily.

- History-taking
- Immunizations
- Patient education
- X-rays
- Laboratory tests
- Reporting by telephone

Know what services you are expected to provide from the different capitation agreements you have with Medicare and Medicaid HMOs. Some plans expect primary care physicians to provide ancillary services, such as X-rays and lab tests. Never contract to provide clinical services you do not feel qualified to do. Although risks are involved, cost-efficiency is the key to succeeding in Medicare and Medicaid HMOs.

Ethical Considerations in Managed Care

The Physician-Patient Relationship

With emphasis on managed care and managed competition, health care reform will greatly increase the concern for ethics in managed care. It is essential that the physician acts to ensure that managed care techniques are implemented in a way that protects patients and the integrity of the physician-patient relationship. By creating conflicting incentives for the physician, some of the techniques of managed care can undermine the physician's fundamental obligation to serve as patient advocate. Moreover, in their zeal to control utilization, managed care plans may inappropriately withhold germane diagnostic procedures or treatment modalities for patients.

At the foundation of the physician-patient relationship is the trust that physicians are dedicated first and foremost to serving the needs of their patients. Without trust, the success of the healing process would be seriously diminished. Physicians are clearly in the best position to know patients' interests, and can advocate within the health care system for patients' needs.

The physician is obligated to provide or recommend treatment when he/she believes that the treatment will materially benefit the patient and not to withhold the treatment to preserve the resources of the managed care plan. Physicians should not engage in bedside rationing. It remains the physician's duty to recommend and to advocate for the patient's right to treatment in any case that would benefit a particular patient.

The decision-making process in patient treatment should include some mechanism for considering the preferences and values of the people whom decisions will most directly affect. Accurate and full disclosure is most important. For example, as part of the process of giving patients informed consent to treatment, physicians should disclose all available treatment alternatives, regardless of cost. This includes those potentially beneficial treatments not offered under the terms of their plan.

It is also critical for managed care plans to have a well-structured appeals process through which physicians and patients can challenge the denial of payment for a particular diagnostic test or therapeutic procedure. Such a process should afford the physician an opportunity to advocate on the patient's behalf before the plan's medical or governing board. Appeal mechanisms for treatment payment denials are essential because policy-level allocation decisions can never fully account for all contingencies and will sometimes underserve individual patients. Managed care plans, as institutions, have an ethical responsibility to allow patients to challenge treatment decisions that directly affect their health and well-being.

In some circumstances physicians have an obligation to initiate appeals on behalf of their patients. Cases may arise in which a health plan has an allocation guideline that is generally fair but in particular circumstances results in unfair denials of care, i.e., denial of care that would materially benefit the patient. In such cases, the physician's duty as patient advocate requires that the physician challenge the denial and argue for the provision of treatment in the specific case. Cases may also arise in which a health plan has an allocation guideline that is generally unfair in its operation. In such cases, the physician's duty as patient advocate requires not only a challenge to any denials of treatment from the guideline but also advocacy at the health plan's policy making level to seek elimination or modification of the guideline.

Conflicts Between Physician and Patient

First, physicians are given incentives to reduce costs of medical care, which could result in longer than prudent delays in treatment, avoidance of certain diagnostic tests, or refraining from an expensive referral. Such incentives may cause patients to wonder whether they are receiving all necessary care or if the monetary concerns are taking precedence.

Physicians must place patients' interest ahead of their own, including financial remuneration. Financial conflicts are inherent in the practice of medicine, regardless of the system of delivery, and physicians generally have been able to maintain their duty to patient welfare despite those conflicts. However, incentives to limit care are more problematic than incentives to provide care.

In general, the stronger of the incentive, the more likely it will create a serious conflict of interest that could lead to less than optimal care being delivered to the patient. The strength of a financial incentive to limit care can be judged by various factors. These include the percentage of the physician's income placed at risk, the frequency of calculations for incentive payments, and the size of the group of physicians being judged for economic performance.

The most effective way to eliminate inappropriate conflicts is to create the use of financial incentives based on quality of outcomes rather than quantity of services delivered. Reimbursement that serves to promote a standard of "appropriate" behavior helps to maintain the goals of professionalism. Unlike incentives based on quantity of services, which penalize the provision of both appropriate and inappropriate services, incentives based on quality of outcomes penalize only inappropriate services.

Judgments about the quality of a physician's practice should be based on the following measures:
- objective outcomes data
- adherence to practice guidelines or other standards of care
- patient satisfaction
- judgment of a physician's peers

Physicians must constantly look for less expensive methods to treat patients. Consulting with other same-specialty physicians to see how they handle similar cases should help.

Patient Autonomy and Responsibility

Patients have a responsibility to make sure they know and understand the terms of their own health care plan. As patient advocates, physicians continue to have duties of disclosure. They must ensure that all treatment alternatives, regardless of cost, are disclosed. They must also ensure that the managed care organization has fulfilled its obligation to disclose the terms of the benefits package, including all limitations and restrictions, as well as the appeals process.

Patient autonomy does not guarantee the right to have all treatment choices funded. Moreover, patients do not have an unlimited claim to physicians' obligation to provide health care. To fully exercise their autonomy, patients need to be fully informed about the philosophy and goals of managed care. Physicians have a duty to disclose financial incentives, to disclose contractual agreements restricting referral, and to ensure that the managed care plan makes adequate disclosure of the details of the plan to subscribers.

Guidelines

For the reasons described above, the AMA Council on Ethical and Judicial Affairs has issued the following guidelines:

- The duty of patient advocacy is a fundamental element of the physician-patient relationship that should not be altered by the system of health care delivery in which physicians practice. Physicians must continue to place the interests of their patients first.

- When managed care plans place restrictions on the care that physicians in the plan may provide to their patients, the following principles should be followed:

    - any broad allocation guidelines that restrict care and choices — that go beyond the cost-benefit judgments made by physicians as a part of their normal professional responsibilities — should be established at a policymaking level so that individual physicians are not asked to engage in ad hoc bedside rationing.

    - Regardless of any allocation guidelines or gatekeeper directives, physicians must advocate for any care they believe will materially benefit their patients.

    - Physicians should be given an active role in contributing their expertise to any allocation process and should advocate for guidelines that are sensitive differences among patients. Managed care plans should create structures similar to hospital medical staffs that allow physicians to have meaningful input into the plan's development of allocation guidelines. Guidelines for allocating health care should be reviewed on a regular basis and updated to reflect advances in medical knowledge and changes in relative costs.

    - Adequate appellate mechanisms for both patients and physicians should be in place to address disputes regarding medically necessary care. In some circumstances, physicians have an obligation to initiate appeals on behalf of their patients. Cases may arise in which a health plan has an allocation guideline that is generally fair but in particular circumstances result in unfair denials of care. An example is denial of care that, in the physician's judgment, would materially benefit the patient. In such cases, the physician's duty as patient advocate requires that the physician challenge the denial and argue for the provision of treatment in the specific case. Cases may also arise in which a health plan has an allocation guideline that is generally unfair in this operation. In such cases, the physician's duty as patient advocate requires not only a challenge to any denials of treatment from the guideline but also advocacy at the health plan's policymaking level to seek an elimination or modification of the guideline. Physicians should assist patients who wish to seek additional appropriate care outside the plan when the physician believes the care is in the patient's best interests.

    - Managed care plans must adhere to the requirement of informed consent that patients be given full disclosure of material information. Full disclosure requires that managed care plans inform potential subscribers of limitation or restrictions on the benefits package when they are considering entering the plan.

- Physicians also should continue to promote full disclosure to patients enrolled in managed care organizations. The physician's obligation to disclose treatment alternatives to patients is not altered by any limitations in the coverage provided by the patient's managed care plan. Full disclosure includes informing patients of all their treatment options, even those that may not be covered under the terms of the managed care plan. Patients may then determine whether an appeal is appropriate or whether they wish to seek care outside the plan for treatment alternatives that are not covered.

- Physicians should not participate in any plan that encourages or requires care at or below minimum professional standards.

■ When physicians are employed or reimbursed by managed care plans that offer financial incentives to limit care, serious potential conflicts are created between the physician's personal financial interests and the needs of their patients. Efforts to contain health care costs should not place patient welfare at risk. Thus, financial incentives are permissible only if they promote the cost-effective delivery of health care and not the withholding of medically necessary care.

- Any incentives to limit care must be disclosed fully to patients by plan administrators on enrollment and at least annually thereafter.

- Limits should be placed on the magnitude of fee withholds, bonuses, and other financial incentives to limit care. Calculating incentive payments according to the performance of a sizable group of physicians rather that on an individual basis should be encouraged.

- Health plans or other groups should develop financial incentives based on quality of care. Such incentives should complement financial incentives based on the quantity of services used.

■ Patients have an individual responsibility to be aware of the benefits and limitations of their health care coverage. Patients should exercise their autonomy by public participation in the formulation of benefits packages and by prudent selection of health care coverage that best suits their needs.

American Medical Association

Preface

The American Medical Association (AMA) defines "managed care" as systems or techniques that are used to affect access to and control payment for health care services. Managed care techniques most often include one or more of the following:

- prior, concurrent, and retrospective review of the medical necessity and appropriateness of services and/or site of services.

- contracts with selected health care professionals or providers;

- financial incentives or disincentives related to the use of specific providers, services, or service sites;

- controlled access to and coordination of services by a case manager; and

- payer efforts to identify treatment alternatives and modify benefit restrictions for high-cost patients (i.e., high-cost case management).

During the past decade, interest in managed care among employers, third party payers, and state and federal legislators has risen steadily, even though the ability of managed care techniques to contain health care costs continues to be debated. As a result, managed care and related strategies are influencing the practice of medicine and exerting immense pressure on physicians. These trends will continue as federal and state health system reform efforts expand and additional managed care mechanisms are introduced.

The AMA strongly believes that the needs of patients are best served by free market competition and free choice by physicians and patients between alternative delivery and financing systems, with the growth of each system determined not by preferential regulation and subsidy, but by the number of persons who prefer that mode of delivery or financing. Currently, many patients have limited choice of health plans offered by their employers and their access to physicians under these plans often is restricted as well. As a result, the AMA believes that all health plans, especially those that utilize closed panels that restrict a patient's choice of physician, should offer patients the option of purchasing a "point of service" rider.

The AMA has continued to develop a strong policy base and has established various mechanisms to address issues related to managed care. Two of these mechanisms, the Managed Care Partnership and the Managed Care Forum, bring together members of the AMA Federation to discuss policy considerations on those managed care issues that directly influence physicians, clinical practice, and patient care. In addition, the AMA offers a series of products and resources to assist physicians in contracting with managed care plans or in forming their own managed care entity.

The following *Principles of Managed Care* represents a key component in these efforts. Issues addressed in the *Principles* include disclosure provisions, selective contracting, financial incentives, case management, physician involvement, and utilization review and management. It is hoped that these principles, which are based entirely on AMA policy, will promote effective managed care techniques that are fair and equitable to physicians in ensuring that high quality health care services are delivered to patients.

Disclosures Provisions

All managed care plans should be required to clearly and understandably communicate to enrollees and prospective enrollees, in a standard disclosure format, those services which they will and will not cover and the extent of that coverage. The information disclosed should include the proportion of plan income devoted to utilization management, marketing, and other administrative costs, and the existence of any review requirements, financial arrangements, or other restrictions that may limit services, referral, or treatment options.

Physicians must disclose any financial inducements or contractual agreements that may tend to limit the diagnostic and therapeutic alternatives that are offered to patients or restrict referral or treatment options. Physicians may satisfy their disclosure obligations by assuring that the managed care plan makes adequate disclosure to patients enrolled in the plan. Physicians must also inform their patients of medically appropriate treatment options regardless of their cost or the extent of their coverage.

Managed care plans or networks that use criteria to determine the number, geographic distribution, and specialties of physicians needed should report to the public, on a regular basis, the impact that the use of such criteria has on the quality, access, cost, and choice of health care services provided to its patients.

It is the responsibility of the patient and his or her managed care plan to inform the treating physician of any coverage restrictions imposed by the plan.

Selective Contracting

Managed care plans or networks should provide public notice within their geographic service areas when applications for participation are being accepted.

Physicians should have the right to apply to any managed care plan or network in which they desire to participate and to have that application approved if it meets physician-developed, objective criteria that are available to both applicants and enrollees and are based on professional qualifications, competence, and quality of care. Any economic criteria used in such selective contracting should be a demonstrated positive relationship to the quality and appropriateness of care and to professional competency.

Managed care organizations or networks may develop and use criteria to determine the number, geographic distribution, and specialties of physicians needed.

Managed care organizations should disclose to physicians applying to the plan the selection criteria used to select, retain, or exclude a physician from a managed care plan, including the criteria used to determine the number, geographic distribution, and specialties of physicians needed.

Selective contracting decisions made by managed care plans should be based on an evaluation of multiple criteria related to professional competency, quality of care, and the appropriateness by which medical services are provided. In general, no single criterion should provide the sole basis for selecting, retaining, or excluding a physician from a managed care plan.

Managed care plans that contract with selected providers should have an established appeals mechanism by which any provider willing to abide by terms of the plan contract could challenge a decision to deny the provider's application for participation in the plan.

All managed care contracts should expressly require the managed care plan to provide meaningful due process protections, in order to prevent wrongful and arbitrary contract terminations that leave the physician without means of redress.

Prior to initiation of actions leading to termination or nonrenewal of a physician s participation contract for any reason, the physician shall be given notice specifying the grounds for termination or nonrenewal, a defined process for appeal, and an opportunity to initiate and complete remedial activities except in cases where harm to patients is imminent or an action by a state medical board or other governmental agency effectively limits the physician's ability to practice medicine.

All "hold harmless" clauses in managed care contracts should be explicitly identified as such. Physicians should consider consulting with legal counsel prior to contracting with a managed care entity to prevent the imposition of unfair liability upon the physician. Physicians should have the right to enter into whatever contractual arrangements with managed care plans they deem desirable and necessary, but should be aware of the potential for some types of plans to create conflicts of interest because of financial incentives to withhold medically indicated services.

Financial Incentives

Financial incentives should be used only if they promote the cost-effective delivery of health care, not the withholding of medically necessary care, and should be developed based on quality of care.

Physicians must not allow financial incentives to influence their judgment of appropriate therapeutic alternatives or deny their patients access to appropriate services based on such inducements. Instead, they must continue to place the interests of their patients first. The duty of patient advocacy is a fundamental element of the physician-patient relationship that should not be altered by the system of health care delivery in which physicians practice.

Physician payments that provide an incentive to limit the utilization of service should not link financial rewards with individual treatment decisions over periods of time insufficient to identify patterns of care, or expose the physician to excessive financial risk for services provided by other physicians or institutions to whom patients have been referred for diagnosis or treatment.

When risk sharing arrangements are relied upon to deter excess utilization, physician incentive payments should be based on performance of groups of physicians rather than individual physicians, and should not be based on performance over short periods of time.

All managed care contracts which include incentive withholds for the payment of physician fees should include provisions for an independent audit to assure timely reimbursement of withholds and that the amount being withheld is appropriate, reasonable, and in keeping with the terms of the contract.

Case Management

With the present specialization of medical services, it is advantageous to have one individual with overall responsibility for coordinating the medical care of the patient; the physician is best suited by professional preparation to assume this leadership role.

Managed care plans should provide enrollees, on an ongoing basis, with the right to select a new primary physician from the panel of physicians, and to appeal to the plan when the patient is dissatisfied with his/her present primary physician.

Managed care plans using the preferred provider concept should not use coverage arrangements which impair the continuity of a patient's care across different treatment settings.

All managed care plans, particularly closed panels that restrict an enrollee's choice of physicians or hospitals, should offer a "point of service" feature so that enrollees may elect to see a physician outside the plan at additional cost to themselves.

The primary goal of high-cost case management or benefits management programs should be to help to arrange for the services most appropriate to the patient's needs; cost containment is a legitimate but secondary objective. In developing an alternative treatment plan, the benefits manager should work closely with patient, attending physician, and other relevant health professionals involved in the patient s care.

Any managed care plan which makes available a benefits management program for individual patients should not make payment for services contingent upon a patient's participation in the program or upon adherence to treatment recommendations.

Physician Involvement

All managed care plans and medical delivery systems must include significant physician involvement in their health care delivery policies similar to those of self-governing medical staffs in hospitals. The principles of self-governance for managed care medical staffs should include, but not be limited to:

- the development of medical staff bylaws which cannot be unilaterally changed by the governing board of the managed care entity;
- physician election of representatives to the governing board and other appropriate committees including credentialing, privileging, quality assurance, and utilization review;
- due process protections for physicians credentialed by the managed care entity; and
- full indemnification by the managed care entity of physicians who, in good faith, serve as members of credentialing, quality assurance, and utilization review committees of the entity.

Physicians participating in managed care plans must be able to comment on, and present their positions regarding, the managed care plan policies and procedures without threat of punitive action.

Utilization Review and Management

The medical protocols and review criteria used by managed care plans in any utilization review of management program must be developed by physicians.

Managed care plans should be required to disclose to physicians, on request, the screening and review criteria, weighting elements, and computer algorithms used in the review process, as well as how they were developed.

Any managed care plan utilizing a prior authorization program should act within two business days on any patient or physician request for prior authorization and respond within one business day to other questions regarding medical necessity of services.

Any managed care plan requiring prior authorization for covered services should provide enrollees subject to such requirements with consent forms for release of medical information for utilization review purposes, to be executed by the enrollee at the time services requiring prior authorization are recommended by the physician.

A physician of the same specialty must be involved in any decision by a utilization review or management program to deny or reduce coverage for services based on questions of medical necessity.

Any physician who makes judgments or recommendations regarding the necessity or appropriateness of services or site of services should be licensed to practice medicine and actively practicing in the same jurisdiction as the practitioner who is proposing or providing the reviewed service, and should be professionally and individually accountable for his or her decisions.

A physician whose services are being reviewed for medical necessity should be provided the identity and credentials of the reviewing physician on request.

Any managed care plan implementing utilization review or management programs should establish an appeals process whereby physicians, other health care providers, and patients may challenge policies for services, and have the right to review any coverage denial based on medical necessity by a physician who is of the same specialty and has appropriate expertise and experience in the field.

Any managed care plan that compiles information on physician performance should share that information with the practitioners involved prior to public release.

Any health plan using managed care techniques should be subject to legal action for any harm incurred by the patient resulting from application of such techniques. Health plans should also be subject to legal action for any harm to enrollees resulting from failure to disclose prior to enrollment any coverage provisions, review requirements, financial arrangements, or other restrictions that may limit services, referral, or treatment options, or negatively affect the physician s fiduciary responsibility to his or her patient.

The principles contained in this publication have been abstracted and summarized from the following:

AMA Policy Compendium, Policies 165.908, 165.909, 285.982, 285.983, 285.984, 285.991, 285.994, 285.995, 285.996, 285.997, 285.998

PRACTICE SUCCESS! SERIES

Exhibits

- *Determine the Weighted Average of the Plan (Schedule A)* 9-1

- *Determine the Weighted Average of the Plan (Schedule B)* 9-2

- *Patient Satisfaction Survey* 10-1

Determine the Weighted Average of the Plan   Exhibit 9-1

SCHEDULE A

CPT Code (A)	Your Fee (B)	McGraw-Hill RVU (C)	McGraw-Hill Conversion Factors (D)	McGraw-Hill Conv. Factors @ $___ (E)	Medicare RVU (F)	RBRVS Ind. Conv. Factors (G)	RBRVS Conv. Factor @ $___ (H)
99201							
99202							
99203							
99204							
99205							
99211							
99212							
99213							
99214							
99215							
99241							
99242							

Determine the Weighted Average of the Plan

Exhibit 9-2

SCHEDULE B

CPT Code	Your Fee	Medicare Allowable	Plan #1		Plan #2		

Patient Satisfaction Survey   Exhibit 10-1

PATIENT SATISFACTION SURVEY

Below are a number of questions about your recent visit to our office. We want to provide the best service possible, but to do so we need to know what we are doing right and what needs improvement. Please take a few minutes to complete this survey and return it to us in the envelope provided. Your opinions are very important to us.

About yourself:

Age: _____   Name (optional): _____   Sex: _____

Address: _____

Marital Status: ❑ Single   ❑ Married   ❑ Widow(er)

Name and Age of Spouse: _____

Names and Ages of Children: _____

Occupation: Yours: _____   Spouse: _____

Education: Yours: _____   Spouse: _____

Best Times for Appointments: _____

Are we the main source of health care for your family?   ❑ Yes   ❑ No

If members of your family are seeing other physicians, please tell us who and why.

Spouse: _____

Children: _____

Other: _____

Type of Insurance:

❑ Blue Cross   ❑ HealthChoice   ❑ Aetna   ❑ Medicare   ❑ Medicaid   ❑ Self-pay   ❑ Other

About Our Physicians:

Which physician did you see? _____

Please tell us how you would rate each of the following:

Scheduling	Excellent	Average	Poor
1. Promptness in which the phone was answered when you called the office			
2. Courtesy of the staff taking your call			
3. Efficiency of staff scheduling your appointment			
4. Availability of appointment times			
Physical Plant	**Excellent**	**Average**	**Poor**
5. Convenience of our location			
6. Ease of parking			
7. Cleanliness and comfort of the office			
8. Cleanliness of the restroom			
Front Office Personnel	**Excellent**	**Average**	**Poor**
9. Courtesy of the receptionist when you arrived at the office			
10. Courtesy and helpfulness of the business personnel			
11. Helpfulness of the staff in explaining your bill and payment responsibilities			
12. Accuracy of your bill			

Front Office Personnel (continued)	Excellent	Average	Poor
13. Helpfulness of the staff with insurance matters			
14. Ease of scheduling follow-up appointment time			
15. Ease of getting questions answered by phone about your bill			
16. Time you waited in the waiting room to see physician — how long? _____			
17. Time you waited in the examination room to see physician — how long?_____			
Doctors	Excellent	Average	Poor
18. Responsiveness and degree of caring the physician showed you			
19. Time spent with the physician? Length of time _____			
20. Explanation by physician of your diagnosis			
21. How clearly did the physician answer your questions			
22. Explanation by physician of any follow-up visits			
23. Explanation by physician of any follow-up procedures			
24. Ability of the physician to communicate in layman s (e.g. understandable) terms			
25. Explanation by physician regarding medications			
26. Explanation by physician regarding test results			
27. Information provided by physician regarding preventive care			
Nurses	Excellent	Average	Poor
28. Attitude and expertise			
29. Respect for your sense of modesty and privacy			
30. Promptness of obtaining test results — who called with results? _____			
31. Ease of getting questions answered by phone about follow-up procedures, medications or test results			
After-Hours and Weekend Care	Excellent	Average	Poor
32. Physician availability after hours			
33. Promptness and courtesy of answering service			
34. Speed with which physician returns your call			

Reason You Decided to Seek Medical Treatment in this Office.

❏ Near home or business ❏ Referral by another patient ❏ Referral by local medical society
❏ Yellow Pages listing ❏ Physician referral service ❏ Physician belongs to my insurance plan
❏ Referral by another physician; who?_____
❏ Other _____

Do you have any other comments or suggestions to help us improve our service to you? _____
_____
_____
_____
_____

PLEASE MAIL YOUR COMPLETED SURVEY IN THE POSTAGE PAID ENVELOPE PROVIDED. THANK YOU FOR TAKING THE TIME TO ANSWER THIS QUESTIONNAIRE. WE LOOK FORWARD TO SERVING YOU AGAIN.

Bibliography

Gaston, J. Harper, M.D., *Managed Care Medicine*, "The Optimal Financial Payment Mechanisms of the Future: Reflections on Ten Years of Experience with Capitation." September, 1995, pages 15-22, 41.

Health Care Quality Improvement Act of 1986, Title IV, Public Law 99-660; 45 Code of Federal Regulations, Part 60, page 111.

Katz, Harvey P. M.D., *Telephone Medicine: Triage & Training—A Handbook for Primary Care Health Professionals.* F. A. Davis Co., 1990.

Lee, David W., Ph.D. *Capitation: The Physician's Guide.* Chicago, IL: American Medical Association, 1995.

Mitchell, Susan, Editor. *Encyclopedia of Health Care Reform Terms,* Allina Health System, Minneapolis, MN. August, 1994, page 594.

Nash, David B., MD. *The Physician's Guide to Managed Care.* Gaithersburg, MD: Aspen Publishers, Inc., 1994.

The Journal of the American Medical Association, "Ethical Issues in Managed Care," Vol. 273, No. 4., pages 330-35, January 25, 1995.

Unland, James J. *A Guide to Forming Physician Directed Managed Care Networks.* Chicago, IL: American Medical Association, 1994.

Vogel, David E. *The Physician and Managed Care.* Chicago, IL: American Medical Association, 1993.

Walker, Lauren M. *Medical Economics,* "Turn Capitation into a Moneymaker," March 13, 1995, pages 58-73.

Wieland, James B. *The Internist's Guide to Negotiating Managed Care Contracts & Capitation Rates.* Washington, DC: American Society of Internal Medicine, 1995.

Winkenwerder, William, MD. *Doctors Resource Service: Primary Care and Specialist Physician Roles in a Managed Care Environment.* Chicago, IL: American Medical Association, 1994.

Woodke, Dale, R.N., N.P. *Telephone Triage Protocols for Primary Care Centers.* American Academy of Family Physicians, (800) 944-0000, refer to item number 90337.

Index

A

Access	12
Accountable Health Plans (AHP)	12
Accredited Capitated Provider (ACP)	12
Actuarial Analysis	12, 67-68
Acute Rehabilitator	28-29
Adjusted Average Per Capita Cost (AAPCC)	87
Administrative Service Only (ASO)	13
Adverse Selection	61
All Payer System	13
Alternative Delivery Systems	13
Alternative Primary Care Practitioner	13
Ambulatory Care	13
Antitrust Laws	13
Appropriate and Necessary Health Services	13
Audit	84-85

B

Bad Debt Expense	14
Balanced Billing	14
Basic Capitation	59
Benchmarking	14
Beneficiary	14
Bonus Payments	63
Bundling	14

C

Canadian Health System	14
Capital Expenditure	14
Capitated Basis	14
Capitation	14-15, 59, 65-69, 88
Capitation for Subspecialists	64
Care Coordinator	18
Care Manager	18
Carve-outs	15, 63
Case Management	100
Case Mix	15
Catchment Area	15
Charity Care	15
Clinical Practice Guidelines	15
Closed Panel	15
Community Rating	15
Consultant	28
Continuous Quality Improvement (CQI)	16
Continuum of Care	16
Contractual Adjustments	16
Copayment(s)	16, 64, 67
Cost Analysis	44
Cost Shifting	16
Cost Effective	16
Cost Benefit Analysis	55
Cost Effectiveness Studies	55
Cost Identification Studies	55
Covered Service	16
Current Procedural Terminology, Fourth Edition (CPT-4)	61

D

Decision Maker	26
Deductibles	64
Direct Contracting	16
Direct Contract Model	10
Disclosures Provisions	98

E

Economic Analysis	55
Educator	26
Employer Buying Federation	16
Encounter Level Data	17
Ethical Considerations	91-94
Evaluator	26
Exclusive Provider Organization (EPO)	7, 17
Experience Rating	17
Expert Diagnostician	28
Explanation of Benefits (EOB)	17, 32
Explanation of Medical Benefits (EOMB)	51

F

Federally Qualified HMO	17
Fee-for-Service	17
Financial Incentives	99
Fiscal Intermediary	17
Fiscal Insolvency	22, 36, 37, 61
501(c)3 Status	17

G

Gag Clause	39
Gatekeeper	18, 25-28
Group Practice Model	8-9
Group Practice Without Walls (GPWW)	7, 18
Group Purchaser	18
Guaranteed Issue	18

H

Health Care Financing Administration (HCFA)	19, 23, 88
Health Care Quality Improvement Act of 1986	111
Health Care Entity	13
Health Maintenance Organization (HMO)	8, 18
Health Outcome	18
Health Promotion and Prevention	18
Health Status	18-19
Hold Harmless	19, 37

I, J, K

Incurred But Not Reported (IBNR)	63
Independent Physicians Association (IPA)	9-10
Independent Practice Association Model	9-10, 19
Independent Practice Association (IPA)	10, 19
Information Sharing	54
Insured Services	19
Integrated Delivery System (IDS)	10, 19
Integrated Provider Network (IPN)	19
Intermediary	17
(IRS) 501(c)3 Status	17

L, M

Long Term Care	20
Managed Care/Managed Care Organizations	1-5, 20
Management Services Organization (MSO)	11, 20
Management Tools	27-28, 29-30
Marketing	75-83
McGraw-Hill	33, 67, 71
Medicaid	20, 87-89
Medical Resource Management	55
Medicare	20, 71, 87-89
Medicare, Part A	20
Medicare, Part B	21, 88
Medicare Supplemental Plans	21
Member Months	21
Midlevel Practitioner (MLP)	21
Multi-hospital System	21

N, O

Navigator	26
Negotiator	26
Network Model	9
No Balance Billing	19
Outcomes Measurement	21
Outcomes Research	21

P, Q

Panel Size	61
Patient Advocate	91-93
Patient Satisfaction	77-78, 82-84, 109-110
Peer Review Organization	21
Percentage of Premium Reimbursement	64
Personal Care Manager	27
Physician Education	53
Physician-Hospital Organization (PHO)	11, 22, 37
Physician-Patient Relationship	91-94
Physician Involvement	100
Point of Service Plan (POS)	11
Practice Guidelines	54
Practice Parameters	22
Preexisting Condition	22
Preferred Provider Organization (PPO)	11, 22, 37
Primary Care	22
Quality Assurance	34, 38

R

Rehabilitator	28
Reinsurance	22
Relative Value Scale (RVS)	33, 67, 71
Relative Value Unit Scale (RVUS)	69, 71
Repricer	22
Resource Based Relative Value Scale (RBRVS)	23, 71
Risk Adjustment	23
Risk Pools	61-62
Risk Withhold	23

S

Selective Contracting	98-99
Self-Insured Companies	22
Shared Risk Services	23
Specialists' Roles	28-29
Specialty HMO Models	10
Staff Model	8
Stop-Loss	23

T-Z

Third Party Administrator (TPA)	23, 68
Third Party Payer	23
Total Quality Management	23
Triple Option Plan (TOP)	12, 24
Utilization Management	24
Utilization Review	24, 34, 38, 101
Value	4, 24, 71-73
Weighted Average	72-73, 105-107
Withholds	63, 68